Contents

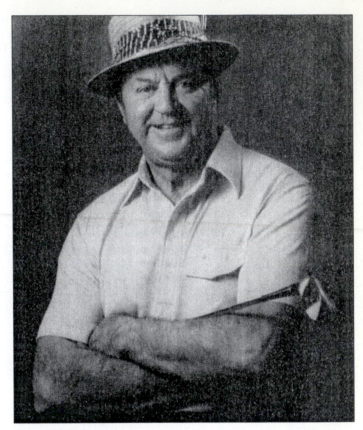

Sam Snead

Golf Professional

Foreword

I have been playing golf for nearly sixty years. Because of my love of the game, I have been able to travel the world over, make a pretty good living, and have a great deal of enjoyment. It is the enjoyment of the challenge of the game and the union with the great outdoors that makes golf the relaxing but invigorating experience that it is.

I learned the game by watching players when I was a caddie. You can learn from professional teachers. With the aid of this textbook, which is the finest I have ever seen, you can learn quickly and correctly. By concentrating on what you need to know, then practicing conscientiously, you can learn this great game effectively and have a whale of a lot of fun for the next forty or fifty years.

When I was young I was a pretty good football player. I ran a good hundred-yard dash, too—about a ten flat. I even played tournament tennis at one time. But golf was the game that captured my imagination and made my life.

As you learn to play better and better I'm sure you'll find, as I have, that golf is the greatest of the lifetime sports. Have fun!

Wadsworth's Physical Education Series

Aerobics Today, by Carole Casten and Peg Jordan

Aqua Aerobics Today, by Carol Casten

Badminton Today, by Tariq Wadood and Karlyne Tan

Golf Today, 2nd edition, by J. C. Snead and John L. Johnson

Jazz Dance Today, by Lorraine Person Kriegel and Kim Chandler-Vaccaro

Racquetball Today, by Lynn Adams and Erwin Goldbloom

Strength Training Today, 2nd edition, by Bob O'Connor, Jerry Simmons, and Pat O'Shea

Swimming and Aquatics Today, by Ron Ballatore, William Miller, and Bob O'Connor

Tennis Today, 2nd edition, by Glenn Bassett, William Otta, and Christine Shelton

Volleyball Today, 2nd edition, by Marv Dunphy and Rod Wilde

The Series Editor for Wadsworth's Physical Education Series

Dr. Bob O'Connor received his B.S. and M.S. degrees in physical education from UCLA and his doctorate from U.S.C. His 40-year teaching experience includes instruction in physical education courses for tennis, weight training, volleyball, badminton, swimming, and various team sports, as well as classes in teaching methods. Internationally, Dr. O'Connor has been an advisor to several Olympic programs in weight training and swimming. He was among the first to popularize strength training for all athletic events. Dr. O'Connor has written extensively in the fields of physical education and health.

Preface

This second edition of *Golf Today* is designed to assist golfers at every level to learn and improve their game. It teaches the beginner the proper grip, stance, and swing. It teaches the intermediate player how to correct errors in the swing and to employ a bit of golf strategy. And it teaches the advanced player more about strategy and how to develop special skills such as reading the greens.

But there is more! Since golf is both a physical and a mental game, a chapter is included on mental practice, detailing the techniques that world-class athletes use daily. Beginners and advanced players alike can practice their golf skills mentally.

As for the physical aspect of golf, it requires more than the ordinary physical conditioning necessary to function in life's daily tasks. When you ask your body to perform an athletic movement as complicated as the golf swing, it must be prepared to deliver strength and flexibility in areas not usually called on. Therefore, a series of stretching and strengthening exercises are presented in this book. In this second edition, we have included chapters on more effective eating and weight control. The two major factors in living a long and effective life are plenty of exercise—and golf certainly qualifies—and proper nutrition. By adding these chapters we believe we have given the reader a much more complete basis for health and fitness.

Every known device for helping every student of the game is included here. There are checklists to help you learn the skills, the rules, and the strategies that will improve your game. There are photographs and drawings that will help you "see" what you have been reading. Thus, we present what we hope is the best possible book for helping you to improve your health and enjoy this wonderful game of golf.

Acknowledgments

The development of this text could not have progressed without helpful criticism and suggestions from colleagues. We gratefully acknowledge the reviewers of this edition: Paul Finnicum, Arkansas State University; Jonathan Nelson, Northern Michigan University; and Sanford Simpson, University of California at Davis. We would also like to acknowledge our colleagues who reviewed the first edition: Steve Dixon, University of Florida; Jim Gilmore, Ohio University; Geraldine Greenlee, Illinois State University; Carolyn Lehr, University of Georgia; Dan Mason, Texas Tech University; William Podoll, Central Michigan University; and Manny Trevino, Moorpark College.

Grateful thanks to Christine Wells for her input in the nutrition, diet, and mental conditioning chapters. Her extensive work in these areas has been a major contribution to this book.

We are also grateful to Christine O'Connor for contributing the chapter on the mental aspect of the sport. This chapter provides information for the reader that, when applied, will enable him or her to maximize their potential.

We cannot thank Christine Kranzler enough for her photography. Her knowledge of sports photography was a great help to us.

Additionally, the authors would like to thank Chris Lehmann for agreeing to model her excellent swing in Chapter 4 on the stance and swing. A former LPGA and European Tour player, she is currently a teaching professional at Westlake Golf Course in Westlake, California. Special thanks are also due to Jorge Badel, teaching professional at Los Verdes Golf Course in Palos Verdes, California for his help in arranging the photo session.

So, for the love of golf—read on and play on.

J. C. Snead
John L. Johnson

1 *The Game of Golf*

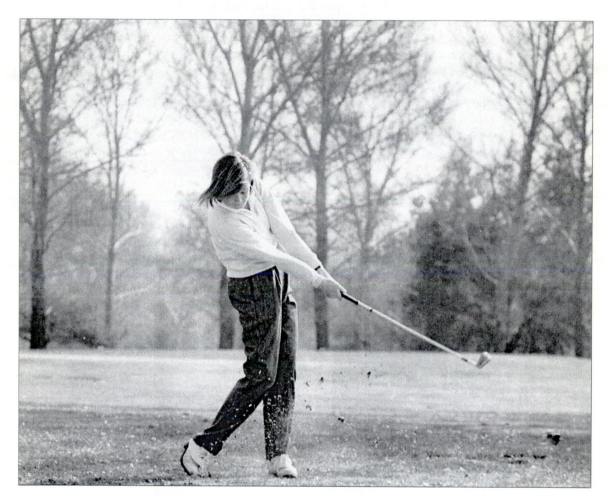

Outline

It has been said that golf is a physical game from the tee to the green but a mental game on the green. It is the mental character of the game that makes it so fascinating. Each course, each hole, and each shot bring you a new challenge. As these challenges are experienced, more and more people are taking up this great game. Today, 27 million Americans now play golf.

Every time you play, you will hit some good shots and some bad ones. The good shots will make you think that you have finally mastered this game. The bad shots will make you wonder if you will ever play well. One of golf's living legends, Ben Hogan, once said that he seldom hit more than five good shots per round. So don't get discouraged. It is a game like life—with ups and downs, troubles and pleasures. It is the complete game.

On the surface the game seems so easy, yet no one has ever played a perfect game of golf. Patience is essential as you learn to tolerate your lack of perfection. Get used to being humbled by the course, the weather, and your lack of perfection—and enjoy the exhilaration of the out-of-doors, your friendly companions, and the enchantment of the game. Take the game as it comes, realizing, as one golf enthusiast has said, that the good shots are accidents and the bad shots are good exercise.

History of Golf

The history of the game may go back to the times of the Romans 2,000 years ago. Some variation of today's game has been played in Europe since that time. And while the Dutch claim to have invented and named it, it is the Scots who developed it into the game we know today.

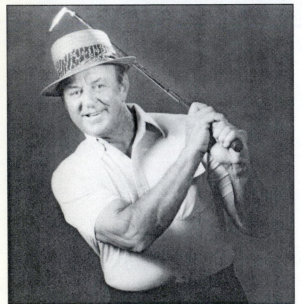

Sam Says

"It's a game where you have to play your foul balls."

In Scotland the game has been played for over 500 years. It started amid turmoil and was banned several times in the early days because it was becoming more popular than archery—and archery practice was needed to defend the country. At the revered St. Andrew's Golf Club in Scotland, the rules became standardized in 1754. But tournaments were not introduced for more than a hundred years.

How Golf Is Played

The game is played over 18 *holes*. Each hole starts from a *tee area*. The objective is to get the ball into a hole on the *green*. And between the tee and the green is the *fairway*.

The tee area may have two or three tees, the closest to the green being the *women's tee*. Women are given a slight advantage because the average woman does not hit the ball as far as the average man. The *men's tee* is farther from the green than the women's tee. Additionally, at many courses there are *championship tees*, which are farther back than the men's tees.

The fairway may be straight or curved (called a *dogleg*). It may be narrow or wide. It may be uphill, downhill, or both. The fairway may be bounded by *rough* (tall grass and bushes), trees, or water. And hazards such as *bunkers* (sand traps), ponds, streams, or trees may impede your progress to the green.

The green is an area covered by closely mown grass and may be bordered by a *fringe* of slightly longer grass. The green may be flat, sloping, or gently rolling. The rolling shots that the golfer uses on the green are called *putts*.

The cup, or *hole*, is marked by the *pin* (flag). The hole is often moved to give the golfer a different challenge each time he or she plays. In major tournaments the holes may be moved daily.

The tee areas

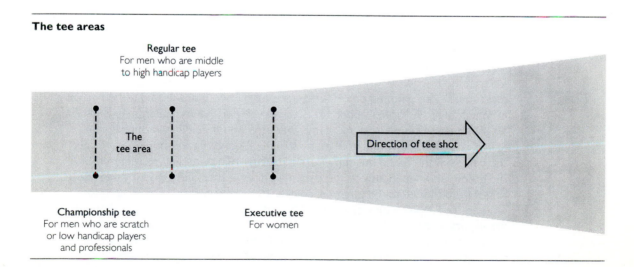

Regular tee
For men who are middle
to high handicap players

The
tee area

Direction of tee shot

Championship tee
For men who are scratch
or low handicap players
and professionals

Executive tee
For women

A typical hole and hazards facing the golfer

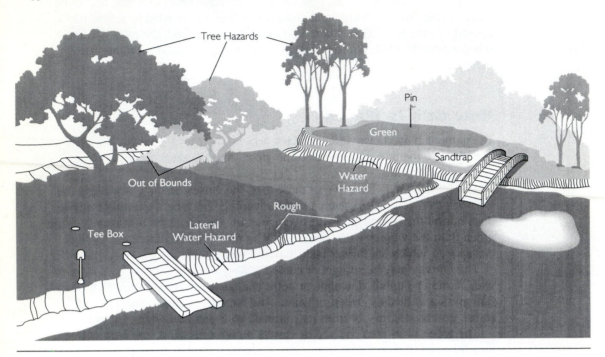

Scoring

Scoring is done by counting the strokes. The person with the least number of strokes wins. Most matches are played over 18 holes, called a *round*, with the total number of strokes counted to determine the winner. This is called *stroke* or *medal* play, and it is almost universally used on the professional tour. Sometimes, however, a match is played on a hole-to-hole basis, called *match play*. The number of strokes on each hole is counted to determine the winner for each hole, and the winner of the tournament is the one who has won the most holes. The winning player who is ahead by two holes is said to be two up in match play. His or her opponent is said to be two down. Match play is used on the much acclaimed "skins" game that appears on television once a year.

Par is a term indicating how many strokes a good player should take to get the ball from the tee to the cup. It assumes that two putts will be required on the green, and depending on the circumstances, either one, two, or three shots to get from the tee to the green. A hole of 250 yards or less for men (210 for women) is a 3-par. Holes of 251 to 470 yards for men (211 to 400 for women) are 4-pars. Longer holes are 5-pars.

Golfers usually speak of their scores in terms of being *over*, *under*, or *even par*. They also have special words to indicate how well they have done on each

Checklist for Establishing Your Handicap

1. Once you have joined a country club or the United States Golf Association, turn in all your 18-hole scores at the pro shops of the golf courses where you play. Sign the scorecard to verify the score.
2. A computerized average of your scores will be used with a formula to determine your handicap. This average will reflect how many strokes you score over par.
3. Your handicap will be posted, in most cases, at your country club or at the club where you belong.
4. You may use this established handicap to play in tournaments or for recreational play.
5. You must keep your handicap current by turning in your scores each time you play.

hole. "I got a par" means you shot whatever that hole's par was—3, 4, or 5. A *birdie* is one stroke under par for that hole. An *eagle* is two strokes under par. A *bogie* is one stroke over par, and a double bogie or triple bogie is two or three strokes over par.

The typical course has 18 holes with a par of 72. This would probably include at least four each of 3-par and 5-par holes, with the remaining holes being 4-pars.

Handicaps are often calculated for better golfers to give them a relative idea as to how well they play. In a tournament, the higher-handicap golfers are given some advantages to equalize their opportunity to win.

The best golfers are called *scratch* golfers and have no handicap. A 2-handicap golfer should average two shots more per round than a scratch golfer. A 36-handicapper would be expected to be 36 strokes higher in score than a scratch golfer.

If handicap players play in a tournament in which the handicaps are used, their handicaps are subtracted from their gross score to give them their net score. So if a scratch golfer shoots a 78, a 2-handicapper shoots a 79, and a 36-handicapper shoots 108, the 36-handicapper will win.

To explain: Since the scratch golfer has no handicap to subtract from the *gross score* of 78 (par being 72), the round puts the scratch golfer six strokes over par. The 79 of the 2-handicapper is reduced by 2 to 77, placing that golfer only five strokes over par. But the 36-handicapper is allowed to subtract 36 strokes from the 108 gross, for a net score of 72, even with par.

Typical scorecard

MEN'S RATING: ☐ BLUE 68.8		WHITE 66.7				RED 64.8				
BLUE COURSE		480	162	392	351	382	190	441	155	490	3043
WHITE COURSE		470	155	375	316	360	165	437	145	475	2898
PAR		5	3	4	4	4	3	4	3	5	35
STROKE HOLE		7	13	3	9	5	15	1	17	11	
Bob	HDCP	5	3	5	5	4	2	4	4	5	37
Chris		5	3	4	4	3	3	4	3	4	33
HOLE		1	2	3	4	5	6	7	8	9	OUT
STROKE HOLE		7	17	3	11	1	13	9	15	5	
PAR		5	3	4	4	4	3	5	3	5	36
RED COURSE		425	130	356	285	340	131	420	133	450	2670

KEEP ALL CARTS AWAY FROM TEES AND GREENS–PLEASE REPLACE DIVOTS

The *scorecard* provides a great deal of information. It will tell you:

- The distance and design of each hole
- The par for each hole
- The par for the course for men and women
- The handicap ranking of each hole

Handicap ranking means that the most difficult hole is ranked as 1 and the least difficult as 18. If you are a 1-handicap player, you will be able to reduce your score by 1 on a hole ranked 1. If you are a 6-handicapper, you will be able to reduce your scores by 1 on *each of the six most difficult holes*. If you are a 22-handicapper, you will be able to reduce your scores by 2 on each of the two toughest holes and by 1 on each of the others.

Typical scorecard—continued

LADIES' RATING: ☐ BLUE 74.8   ☐ WHITE 73.0   ☐ RED 69.5

1	2	3	4	5	6	7	8	9	OUT	TOT		
400	192	488	371	617	405	187	455	210	3325	6368		
378	173	472	330	573	373	140	407	182	3028	5926		
4	3	5	4	5	4	3	4	3	35	70		
6	16	10	12	2	8	18	4	14				
5	3	6	6	5	4	4	5	4	42	79		
4	3	5	5	5	4	2	4	3	35	68		

10	11	12	13	14	15	16	17	18	IN	TOT	ADJ	NET
6	16	2	12	4	10	18	8	14				
4	3	4	4	5	4	3	4	3	34	70		
357	160	390	302	525	340	114	375	163	2726	5396		

PLEASE REPAIR BALL MARKS ON GREENS AND RAKE SAND TRAPS

✔ *Checklist for Keeping a Scorecard*

1. Know how each hole is rated in terms of difficulty. See the rating on your scorecard (see sample scorecard).
2. Note the handicap hole with a checkmark on the scorecard. For example, if you have a handicap of 12, and your opponent has a handicap of 14, your opponent can subtract one stroke on the two highest-handicap holes. (Holes 7 and 14 on the sample scorecard are the two highest-handicap holes for men, and holes 5 and 12 are the two highest-handicap holes for women.)
3. Circle the winning score for each hole.
4. Give yourself a +1 if you win the hole, −1 if you lose it, and E if it is even. (This marking is used by those playing match play or for those who wager on the holes.)
5. Check the scorecard for local rules that allow relief from certain obstacles.

Getting Ready to Play

Arriving at the Course

Upon arrival at the course, you check in at the pro shop to pay your *greens fees*. (On busy courses you should call ahead for reservations.) The pro will tell you your *tee-off* time. You can take some time practicing your shots at the driving range or your putting on the putting green. You will want to be well warmed up before you tee off.

On the Tee

At the tee area, each player should identify the name and number of the ball he or she will use (Titlist 2 or Maxfly 1, for example). This way, players can help locate each other's balls on the course.

On the tee area, you can warm up and take some practice swings until the first player is ready to tee off. Then be quiet and motionless, because the golf swing requires the utmost in concentration.

After the Tee Shot

The player farthest from the hole hits the next shot after the tee shots. This order of play holds true until everyone has completed the hole, or *holed out*. The person with the lowest score then "has the honors" of teeing off on the next hole.

As you play the course, you are required to play the ball *as it lies*. This is one of the challenges of the game. Tall grass, sand, and water are all part of the problems that the course presents. There are some situations in which you are permitted to move your ball, but these may incur a penalty. These situations will be covered in the chapter on rules.

Why Women and Men Play Golf*	Female	Male
To play well	74%	59%
Because spouse plays	60	8
To spend more time with family	42	20
To score well	31	42
The challenge	31	64
To meet people	26	17
The competition	15	45

*(From the National Golf Foundation)

Summary

1. Golf is an enjoyable, challenging, social game that allows a person to compete against himself or herself or against others. It is a game that lets us get back to the beauty of nature while we feel the beauty of our inner nature in the smoothness of the swing.

2. As we examine what has been called "the ancient and royal game," we should realize that playing golf can be fun the first time out. And the joy of playing can be experienced as long as we can swing a club. It is truly a lifelong sport.

3. Golf courses usually have 18 holes. Each hole includes a tee area, a fairway, and a green.

4. The scores can be counted in total strokes for all 18 holes (stroke or medal play) or by counting the winner of each hole (match play).

5. Players at different levels of skill can be given a comparable chance of winning through the use of the handicapping system.

6. The person farthest from the pin always plays the next shot.

7. The person who won the last hole tees off first on the next hole.

2 *Equipment and Courses*

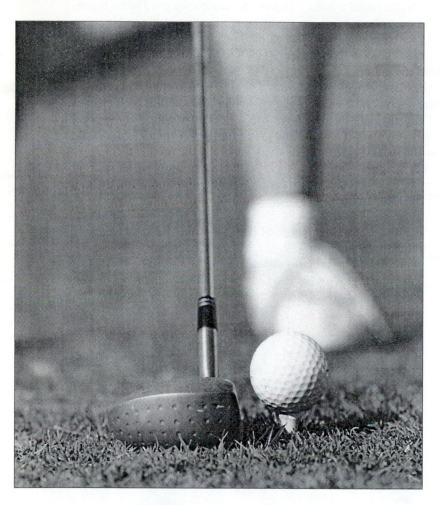

Outline

The Equipment

Golf Clubs

Golf clubs are designed so that with the same swing-speed you can vary the distance and the height that the ball will travel. The parts of the clubs are the *grip*, the *shaft*, and the *head*. The clubs with heavier rounded heads are called *woods*, so named because they used to be made entirely of wood, although now they may be made of various combinations of wood, metal, or other materials. The all-metal clubs with the blade-like heads are called *irons*. The club that is used on the greens to roll the ball toward the hole is called the putter.

The heaviest and longest wood, with a nearly vertical clubface, is the 1-wood, or the *driver*. The 2-wood is slightly lighter and shorter, with a smaller head and a slightly more inclined face. The 3-wood, 4-wood, and 5-wood each have progressively shorter lengths and greater angles of their clubfaces. Being the longest and heaviest club, the driver is generally the most difficult to hit effectively. Each higher-numbered wood is generally slightly easier to control.

The irons are numbered from 1 through 9, with the 1-iron being the longest and having the least amount of clubface angle. Very few nonprofessionals use a 1-iron.

The *pitching wedge* has even more loft than a 9-iron. The sand wedge has even more loft than the pitching wedge. The sand wedge has a very heavy flange, which prevents it from going too deeply into the sand.

Putters come in many shapes and sizes, some with very light heads and some with heavy ones. Shafts may be straight or bent to some degree. The selection of a putter is a highly individual decision.

The average golfer carries 1, 3, and 5 woods

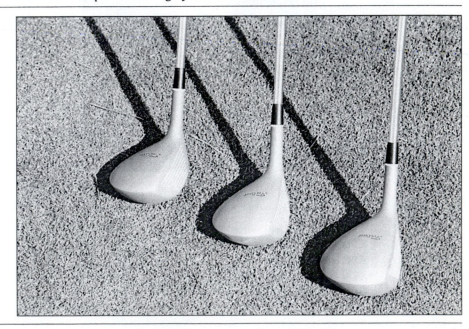

The average golfer carries 3-iron through pitching wedge

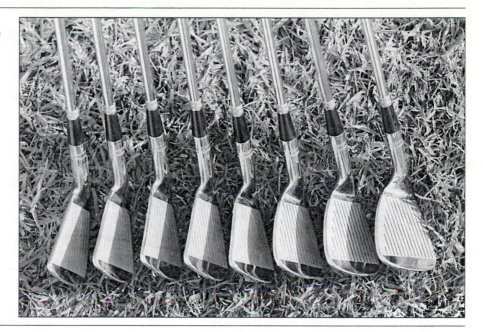

Players are allowed to carry a maximum of 14 clubs. This allows for four woods (the driver and the 2-wood, 3-wood, and 4-wood, or the driver and the 3-wood, 4-wood, and 5-wood), eight irons (usually numbers 2 through 9), a wedge, and a putter. But any combination is possible; for example, you might choose to carry two or three wedges and only two woods. The typical begin-

Putter design varies

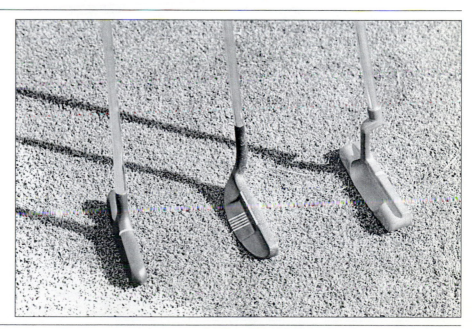

The relative lofts and distances for each club

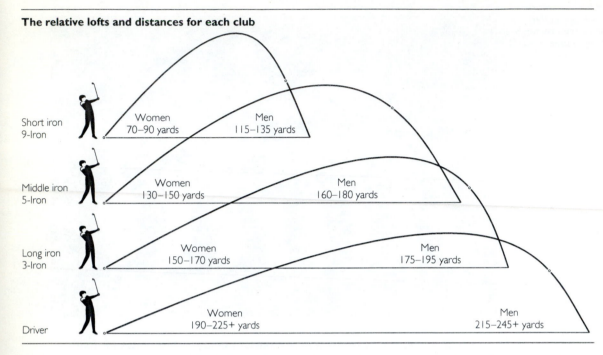

Short iron
9-Iron

Women
70–90 yards

Men
115–135 yards

Middle iron
5-Iron

Women
130–150 yards

Men
160–180 yards

Long iron
3-Iron

Women
150–170 yards

Men
175–195 yards

Driver

Women
190–225+ yards

Men
215–245+ yards

ner's set includes a driver and 3-wood, irons numbered 3, 5, 7, and 9, and a putter.

In buying a set of clubs, it is wise to let a professional assist you. There are some great differences in the clubs. Shaft flexibility is one. The shaft of the club might be very stiff, which allows for more control, or *whippy*, which gives a weaker player more distance with each shot. And there are several variations between these two extremes.

The clubhead

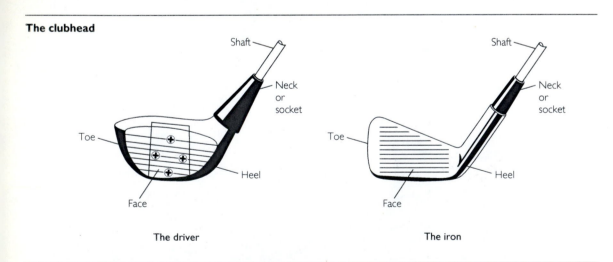

Shaft — Neck or socket

Toe — Heel

Face

The driver

Shaft — Neck or socket

Toe — Heel

Face

The iron

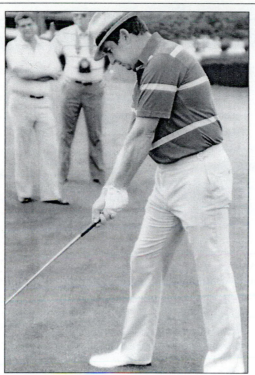

J. C. Says

"This is my twentieth year on the tour, and I have had two good drivers. I wore both of them out and tried to have them repaired, and the club makers ruined both of them."

There are also different swing weights, identified by a letter and number, to tell you how heavy the club will feel as you swing it. A big man might use a D-2 swing weight with a stiff shaft, while a small woman might use a C-8 swing weight with a whippy shaft.

Also, you may have some preconceived notions about clubs that are wrong. For example, tall people do not need longer clubs. They already have enough leverage to hit the ball far. Rather, they need more control. So a tall person might be able to use shorter clubs, whereas a short-armed person might benefit from longer clubs. Grips come in many types and in various materials, including leather and rubber. Find a grip that will not slip in your hands.

It is useful to know the names of the various parts of the clubhead, since these names are often used in teaching. The front of the clubhead is called the *face*. This is the part that comes in contact with the ball. The *sole* is the bottom of the clubhead; it rests on the ground when you are lining up a shot. The *heel* is the part where the shaft of the club joins the head. And the *toe* is the end of the head—opposite the heel.

Golf Balls

Golf balls are available with varying degrees of internal compression. Some have high-compression cores, so will go farther with a powerful swing. Others have low-compression cores, so will go farther when hit with a slower swing. The covers may be very thin or very heavy. Beginners should use tough-covered balls with the *cut-proof* covers. Pros use high-compression balls with thin covers.

Tees

Tees are made of wood or plastic. Wood tees break more easily, but plastic tees can mark the face of the driver. They are not recommended when using new clubs.

Golf Shoes

Officially accepted golf shoes have low heels and rubber spikes. These spikes help to stabilize your feet during the swing. You may be allowed to play in tennis shoes at some courses, but your game will be much improved with real golf shoes.

Golf Clothing

Clothing for playing golf should be comfortable. Knit shirts with collars are typical. Long pants for men and skirts or long pants for women are most commonly accepted. Knee-length shorts are acceptable at most clubs as well, but mini-skirts for women or short-shorts or tee shirts for men or women are banned by many clubs.

Golf Glove

A golf glove is often worn to increase the "feel" of the club and to reduce the chance of perspiration on the hand causing the grip to slip during the swing.

The Golf Course

The average golf course is about 6,000 yards, or a little under 4 miles. Par for 18 holes will generally be 70 to 72 for men, and 73 to 75 for women. There are some short courses, known as *3-pars*, which have nine or eighteen 3-par holes. A more recent innovation is the *executive course*, in which there are a few 4-par holes, but the course is primarily 3-par holes. Unlike the 3-par course, this type of course allows the golfer to use all of his or her clubs during the round.

Golf Holes

The designers of golf courses want to challenge you to hit through narrow areas, over trees and water, and to avoid bunkers and sand traps in the process. They want you to have to putt uphill, downhill, and across a hill. They want to test your skill—and your patience. By knowing the characteristics and the hazards of each hole, you can be better prepared to play it.

Summary

1. Golf clubs vary in length, in weight, and in the *whippiness* (flexibility) of the shaft.

   ■ The longest and heaviest clubs with the large, rounded heads are called woods. They are numbered from 1 (the driver) through 5.

   ■ The shorter clubs with the bladed heads are called irons. They are numbered from 1 through 9.

   ■ The irons with greater loft are called wedges. The most common types of wedges are pitching and sand wedges.

   ■ The club used on the green to roll the ball into the cup is called the putter. There are various designs for putters.

2. Golf balls have different degrees of internal compression, and their covers have varying degrees of toughness.

3. Clothing requirements vary from course to course. Be certain to check on the dress code before arriving at the course.

4. Every serious golfer will wear golf shoes to increase the stability of the stance during the swing.

5. The average golf course is a little under 4 miles.

6. Each hole of a golf course is designed to present a unique challenge.

3 *The Grip*

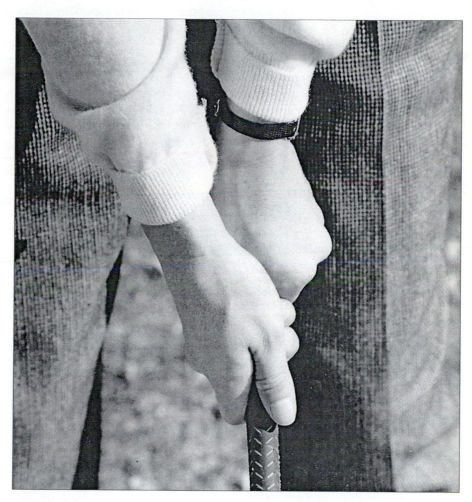

Outline

The Importance of Fundamentals

I t takes a long time and a lot of practice to become a good golfer. Even if you have the athletic ability and the inclination to play well, you still must start with good fundamentals. It doesn't take any talent to grip the club properly and to take the correct stance. Learning the proper swing is what takes the time and the athletic ability.

Anyone who wants to play the game well, especially a beginner, should take lessons. Even the touring pros go to their own professionals for help. You should do the same when you need to improve on some aspect of your game.

People who brag that they never had a lesson and are 15-handicappers often have many problems with their grips and swings. Maybe with proper instruction they could play to a 3 or 4 handicap.

There are four basic parts to the golf swing: your grip, your stance or setup, your backswing (take-away), then your downswing. This chapter will cover the grip. If you miss the grip, all the rest will be wrong.

The Grip

The grip is obviously very important, since it is the contact of your body with the club. If your body swing is to be correctly transmitted to the ball, it must be transmitted through your grip.

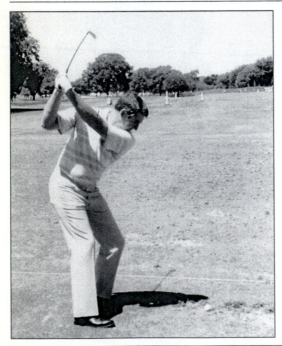

J.C. Says:

"After twenty years on the tour I haven't seen many people with poor fundamentals around. The ones that last are those with solid fundamentals. The old saying on the tour is that those with poor fundamentals may linger, but they won't last."

While there are certain fundamentals for a good grip, there is some room for variation. The grip will become more individualized as you adjust the proper fundamentals to your individual hand size and to the characteristics of your swing.

Most golfers play right-handed. Even left-handed people often find it to their advantage to play right-handed. First, the left-hander's more powerful muscles are on the left side—and this is the side of the body used when swinging right-handed. Second, many courses are set up for right-handers only. Third, there are far more clubs available to the right-handed player. For these reasons, most players play right-handed even if it is not their natural tendency, and, consequently, most of the directions in the book will be for the right-hander.

Step 1: Gripping the Club with the Left Hand

To learn the proper grip, take a club in your left hand, spread your feet to about shoulder width, and put the clubhead on the ground, in front of your left foot with the face of the club square to the way you want to hit the ball. Put your left hand on the club with the back of your hand facing your imaginary target. Put the grip under the meaty part of the heel of your hand behind your little finger. The heel of your hand should be about a half-inch from the end of the club. Now, with your index finger curled lightly around the grip, lift the club up in front of your left hip. You should feel the weight of the club under the heel of

Left-hand grip: Note handle is under heel and cradled in index finger

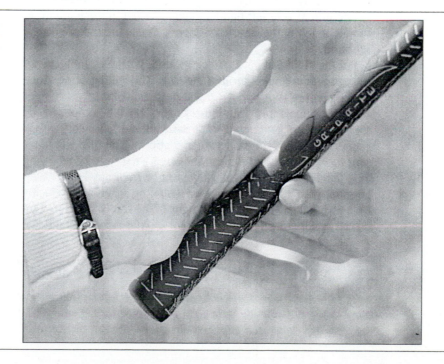

Completed left-hand grip: Club held in last three fingers and across palm

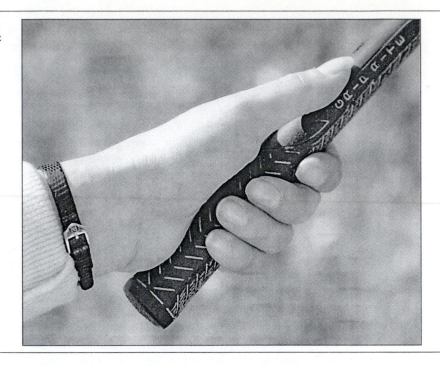

your hand and on the first joint (nearest the palm of your hand) of your index finger. This is the proper feeling of alignment for your grip.

The grip in your left hand shouldn't be felt in the palm of your hand. It should be felt in the last three fingers. These are the pressure points for your left hand.

Put the clubhead back on the ground. With the clubhead still facing the target, wrap your fingers around the club. The feeling of pressure should now be on the palm of your hand in a line perpendicular to your fingers and on your last three fingers (not your index finger). Let it be emphasized that "pressure" does not mean "tightness." Your hand should "connect" with the club, but this connection is not a tight, squeezing grip. A tight grip will tighten the muscles in your forearm and could interfere with a smooth, relaxed swing. One of the all-time famous golfers, Walter Hagen, once said that you shouldn't put any more pressure on a golf club than your would on a pen with which you are writing. Rest your left thumb just to the right of the top of the club. The angle of your thumb and index finger should point to your right shoulder.

Step 2: Gripping the Club with the Right Hand

Your right hand now must connect with your left so that they act as one big hand. Most importantly, your right palm must face the target. This ensures that the club will move in the proper direction—toward the target.

The right hand can be connected to the left three ways

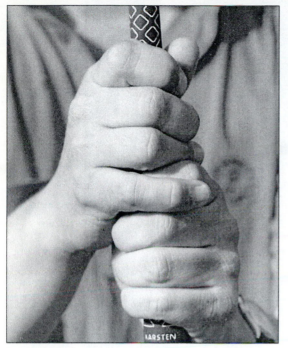

The Vardon grip

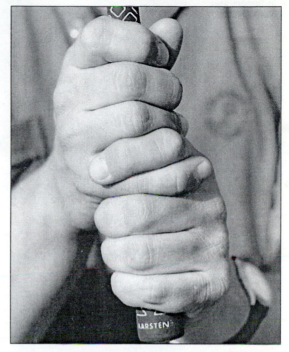

The interlocking grip

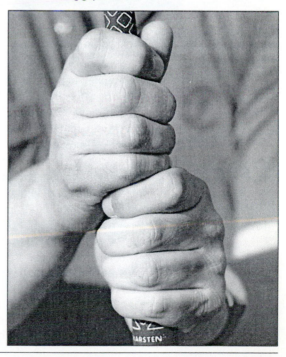

The ten-finger baseball grip

Right-hand grip: Club is held in fingers and right folds over left

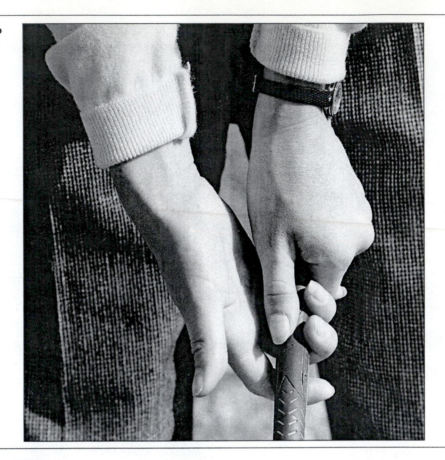

Now you have a choice as to how your right hand will connect with your left to give you the effect of one big hand swinging the club. You have three choices: the overlapping, or Vardon, grip has the little finger of your right hand overlapping the index finger of your left; the interlocking grip has those two fingers crossed over each other; and the ten-finger, or modified-baseball, grip has those two fingers merely touching each other.

Most people prefer the overlapping, or Vardon, grip. It reduces one's chance of having the right hand, which is stronger, control the swing. In this grip, the little finger of the right hand overlaps the index finger of the left hand. The grip is made with the fingers, and the pressure should be felt on the middle and ring fingers of the right hand.

Jack Nicklaus prefers the interlocking grip. Art Wall, who holds the record for most holes-in-one, prefers the ten-finger grip. People with smaller hands often prefer one of these grips.

Now, keeping the palm of your right hand facing the target, roll your right hand over your left thumb. You should now "feel" the club at the base of your fingers on your left hand and the two middle fingers of your right.

The completed grip

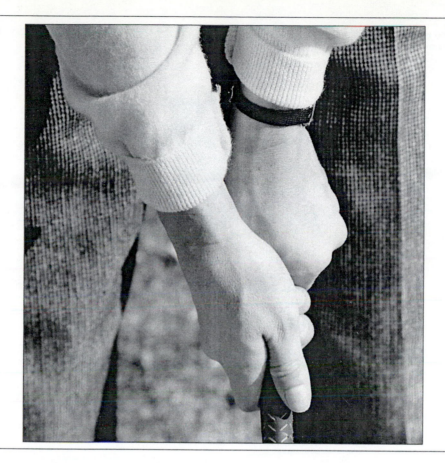

The most common error in the grip is letting the right hand slide under the club. This puts the grip in your right palm. Remember, the pressure should be felt on the *fingers* of the right hand, not on the palm.

Now check the Vs made by the index finger and thumb of each hand. These Vs should both be pointing in the direction of your right shoulder.

A Stronger Versus a Weaker Grip

We have just described the normal grip. Some people like to use a so-called stronger grip (hands moved behind the club—to the right) or a so-called weaker grip (with the hands moved more to the front side of the club—to the left).

A stronger grip allows you to have a weaker swing and still hit straight or to hook the ball left with an average swing. Women who are not particularly strong are more likely to use this grip. But so do many men. In fact, a great many touring pros also use this stronger grip.

A weaker grip requires that you have a strong swing. If you use this grip with a normal or weak swing, you are more likely to slice your shot to the right. Several successful players have used this weaker grip.

The V formed by grip point to area of right shoulder

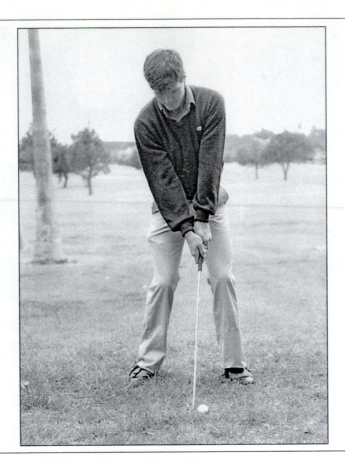

Whichever grip you use, your hands must work together. A strong left hand and a weak right hand, for example, are not going to work together, so you have to adjust one or the other. You might need a pro or golf teacher to help you with this adjustment.

Remember that the grip is there to help you "swing" the club, not to "muscle" it. You're not trying to chop wood or break rocks. So hold the club as if you were holding a bird. That way your arms will stay relaxed and you will be able to swing the club with an easy flowing motion.

Check your grip before you swing. The best car in the world won't run if you don't turn the ignition key. Likewise, you have to have a proper grip in order to transmit power accurately from your swing to the ball.

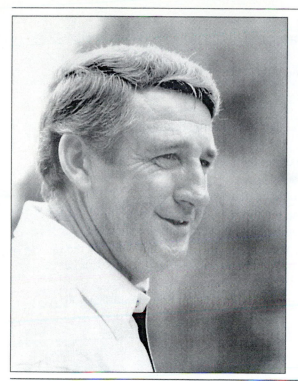

J.C. Says:

"Something you need to look out for is for the pro who thinks there is only one way to teach. The shorter player need a flatter swing. The taller player will be more upright. The "handsy" player may want to stay handsy in the swing. It's difficult for such a player to learn to reduce this hand action. A good teacher finds the way to communicate what is needed. Some people learn better when they see it demonstrated. Some learn better when they move through the motion. Some can key best on a specific part of the body—the left hand, the right hand, the left shoulder or right shoulder, the left knee or the right knee, and so on. A good teacher may have to jump from key to key until finding the one that 'clicks' in the student's mind."

 Checklist for the Grip

1. Your target-side hand (left hand for right-handed golfers) takes a "palm" grip, with the club grip against the fat part of the palm and the thumb slightly to the backside of the grip but pointing straight down the shaft.
2. The right hand takes a "finger" grip.
3. Cover the thumb of your left hand with the palm of your right.
4. Overlap the index finger of your left hand with the little finger of your right hand.
5. The palms of both hands should both face each other.
6. The V of the index finger and thumb of your right hand should point over your right shoulder.
7. Do not grip the club too tightly. Grip it as if you are holding a small bird.
8. Feel and control the club with your left hand.

Summary

1. A golfer's game cannot be stronger than the fundamentals—and the fundamentals start with the grip.

2. The grip is the primary fundamental because it is the connection of the body with the club.

3. In the proper grip:

   - The back of your target hand (left hand for right-handers) must face the target.
   - The club should be gripped under the meaty part of your target (left) hand.
   - The pressure of the club should be near your fingers.
   - Your left thumb should be on the top right of the club with the V angle of your index finger and thumb pointing over your right shoulder.
   - If you are using the popular Vardon grip, the right palm will face the target, and the little finger of the right hand will overlap the index finger of the left hand.
   - You should feel some pressure on the middle and ring fingers of your right hand.

4   *Stance and Swing*

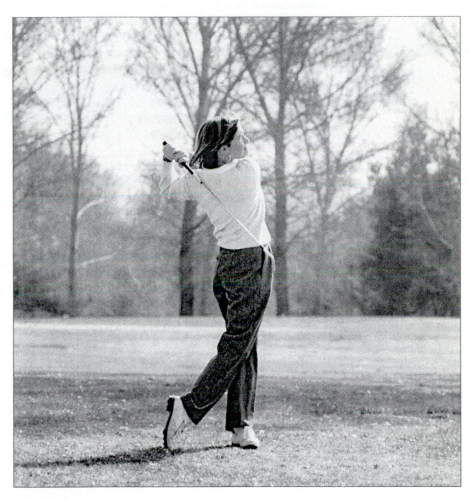

Outline

The Stance

Foot Position

Your stance will vary depending on whether you are taking a full swing or making a short, less powerful *chip* shot to the green. Even on a full shot, your stance may vary depending on whether you want to impart spin to the ball and make it move right (*slice*) or left (*hook*).

If you are on the tee, you will want maximum power, so the inside of your heels should be at least the width of the outside of your shoulders. The foot farther from the target (the right foot for right-handers) should be square to an imaginary line drawn to the target, and the foot nearest the target (left foot for right-handers) should be turned slightly toward the target.

If you drop your target foot (left foot for right-handers) back, you are *opening* your stance. This will make you more likely to slice the ball to the right. If you close your stance by putting your target foot forward, you are more likely to hook the ball to the left.

The shorter the shot, the more you can bring your feet together and drop your target foot (left foot for right-handers) back and open your stance. The more you open your stance, the less power you will have.

Body Position

With your feet spread and your weight on the inside edges of your heels, "sit down" a little by bending your knees slightly, then press your knees inward a bit to aid in your turning action. Then "bow to the ball" by bending slightly at the waist while keeping your upper back straight. From this body position, your arms should hang down naturally from your shoulders. If your hands are too close to your body, your swing will be cramped and stiff.

The three basic stances

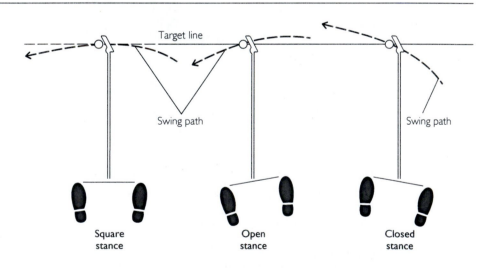

Target line

Swing path

Swing path

Square stance   Open stance   Closed stance

The correct posture at address and three common faults

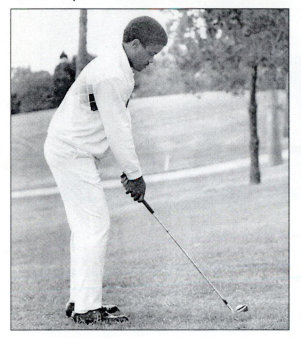

Correct posture: Arms hang naturally and waist is bent

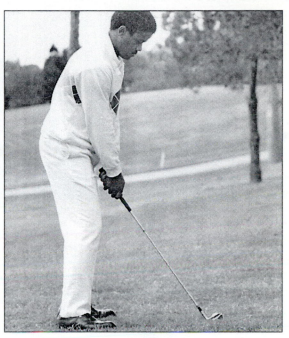

Common fault: No bend at waist and hands too close to body

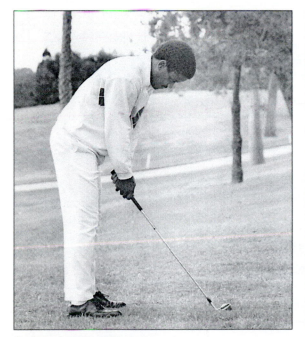

Common fault: Too much bend at waist

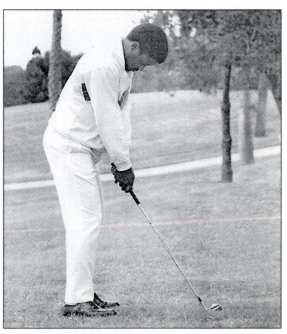

Common fault: Head buried in chest

The correct setup for driver and iron

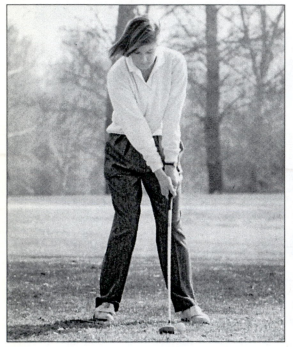

Driver: Use wider stance

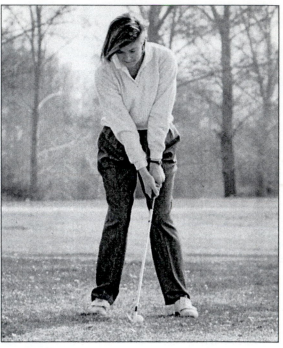

Iron: Use shorter stance

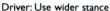

✔ *Checklist for Taking Your Stance*

1. Set your feet apart by approximately the width of your shoulders.
2. Flex your knees so that you are comfortable, then press your knees inward so that you can "set your base."
3. Assume a "semi-sitting" position, and keep your weight evenly distributed on both feet.
4. Think of concentrating your weight on the inside edges of your feet.
5. Your back should be straight, but you should be bending from the waist.
6. Keep your head over the ball and point your chin at the ball so that your shoulder can turn under your chin on the swing.
7. Keep your left arm straight. Feel that the club is an extension of your left arm.
8. Your right shoulder should be lower than your left, because your right arm has to reach farther for the ball.

There should be a straight line from the ball, through the club shaft, your target-side arm (left) and shoulder. Your chin should be pointed, "aimed," at the ball, not buried in your chest.

Setting Up to the Ball

Where you align your feet in relation to the ball depends on your swing and the club you are using. Since each club has a slightly different length (the driver being the longest, followed by the 2 through 5 woods, then the 1 through 9 irons, and finally the wedges, which are the shortest), you will have to set up to the ball slightly closer for each progressively shorter club.

Where you align to the ball in terms of forward and backward placement depends on your swing and the flexibility of the shaft of your club. The clubface should be exactly perpendicular to the desired line of flight of the ball. As a beginner, you might start with the ball directly between your feet. If you find that the ball is going to the right, you can move it farther forward in your stance until your clubface is contacting the ball squarely, and your shot is going straight. More advanced players who are getting a good weight shift will generally play the ball in front of their left heels.

Since the club lengths vary, the clubheads will strike the ball in slightly different parts of the arc of the swing. For this reason, you may find that you will have more success if you set the ball slightly farther away from the target for each shorter club. But as a beginner, you should never set up to the ball farther back than the middle of your stance.

The width of your feet should also vary slightly with each shorter club. They should start wide for the driver and come slightly closer together with each progressively shorter club.

When you set up to the ball, your shoulders and the line of your toes, knees, and hips should be parallel to the direction in which you want the ball to go. So if you are hitting the driver, the line of your shoulders and feet should be down the left edge of the fairway. When you are ready to take the club back, if you look over your shoulder at the target, you should see the target directly over your shoulder or slightly in front of it. The target should never be behind your shoulder.

The Swing

Address and Waggle

In your address position, you should have the feeling of ease, comfort, and relaxation. If you feel tense when you are addressing the ball, you are probably standing too close or too far away. You should feel comfortable at every address. So when you position the ball, don't reach too much—this creates tension in the forearms. Second, don't bend at the waist excessively. This reduces your ability to use your hips in the swing. Find the happy medium where you are not too far from or too close to the ball.

Check to make certain that the bottom (sole) of the club is perpendicular to the line of flight that you desire. Don't align the top of the club with the projected flight because it will not give you a true picture.

Keep your weight behind the ball; that is, the ball should be forward in your stance. Beginners often creep forward on the ball until the ball is almost off their right foot. When this happens, you can't shift your weight properly, and you will probably have to fall away from the ball to hit it because your body is already past the ball before your club can find it.

When you are set up, the shoulder farther from the target (the right shoulder for right-handers) should be lower than your target-side shoulder. This is because the hand away from the target (right hand) is lower on the club, and you therefore have to reach farther since the ball is in front of your target-side (left) heel.

As you are ready to swing, you may want to *waggle* your club. Most golfers do. The waggle is a slight movement of the wrists that moves the clubhead from behind the ball nearly to the ball. This movement is done to reduce tension and to rehearse the wrist action that will occur in a few seconds when you make your complete swing.

 Checklist for Addressing the Ball

1. If you are plying an iron, make sure that your hands are ahead of the ball.
2. If you are playing a wood, your hands should be even with the ball.
3. If you are playing an iron, play the ball from the middle of your stance to the inside of your left heel.
4. If you are playing a wood, play the ball on the inside of your left heel.
5. The ball should not be so far away that you have to "look out" at your hands. You should be able to "look in" at them.
6. Point your chin at the back of the ball.
7. Don't bury your head between your shoulders. Leave room to allow your shoulders to turn easily around your head.

Set the club right in the middle of the ball, and take two or three waggles. This will give you a starting point for your swing and keep the tension out of your arms and wrists. Most good players develop a routine for setting up and taking their waggles. One of the things a waggle accomplishes is to keep you in motion in the address position. Stay in motion. Start with a forward press, then go.

Backswing or Take-Away

In a properly aligned stance, your two arms and the club will make a Y-shape. Keep that Y through the backswing and the downswing.

Take the club away with your target-side (left) shoulder. Keep your upper arm connected to your chest. It is helpful to watch your target-side (left) shoulder to see how far it moves. The eye closest to the target (left eye for right-handers) should see the point of your shoulder at least until it is even with the ball, and preferably until it is behind the ball. How far you can take it back depends on your flexibility.

If your knees have the proper inward bend, they will prevent you from sliding to the right instead of turning your body as you should. And as you complete the coil of your backswing, you will feel that you are braced against your right leg.

The backswing

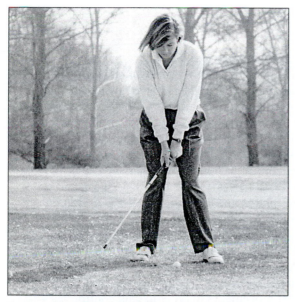

Keep your left shoulder connected to your chest

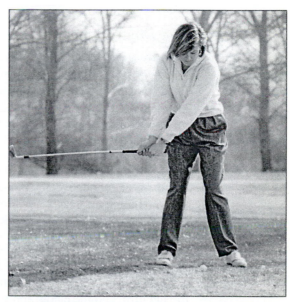

Brace against your bent right leg

The backswing—continued

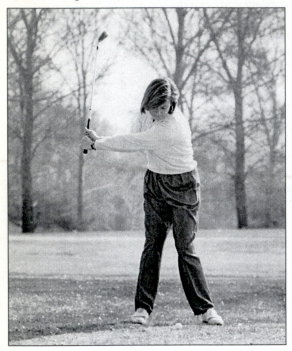

Maintain Y throughout backswing

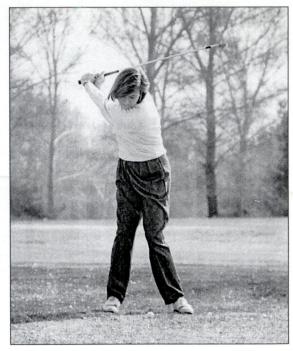

Club does not go beyond parallel at top

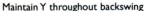

The Downswing

Whether pitching or batting in baseball, hitting a serve in tennis, or teeing off in golf, every basic athletic movement is similar. They all start with a weight shift to the forward leg, then the hips turn, then the shoulders, then the elbows, then the wrists. If you were looking for maximum power, such as in baseball throwing or hitting, you would use all of these joint actions. But as you desire control, such as in a tennis ground stroke or a golf shot, you eliminate one or more of these movements.

For example, a baseball player pitching or a tennis player serving use all of the above-mentioned joints in their motion. But while the pitcher takes a big step in shifting his weight, the tennis player just leans into the serve to shift that weight. A golfer leans even less in the weight shift.

Furthermore, to eliminate potential errors, the beginning tennis player will not use the wrist or elbow in the forehand stroke. The golfer will eliminate left elbow bend for the same reason. And in the shorter, more controlled golf strokes, such as chipping and putting, the golfer may eliminate the weight shift, the hip turn, and the elbow and wrist movements in order to gain control.

Even in the most powerful golf swing, control is of utmost importance. The golfer therefore will not step with the forward foot, nor bend the left arm, nor hit hard with the wrists. Control is more important than power.

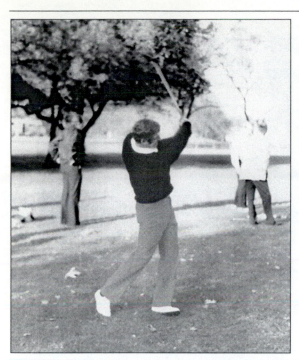

J.C. Says:

"I never felt comfortable taking a lesson from somebody who told everybody the same thing. For example, I can relate to my right shoulder or my left shoulder, but somebody else may relate to his hips. I often use illustrations, such as throwing the ball underhand or throwing dirt into a truck by the shovelful. If you are throwing the dirt up, you will shift your weight forward, but some golfers can't relate to manual labor. It's always more difficult for me to teach them. I just don't know how to relate drinking tea to a golf swing. It is a game of opposites. That is what makes it so difficult."

The golf swing starts with the legs, with a push from the inside of the rear foot (right foot for right-handers). You will feel the muscles contract in the top of the inside edge of your thigh as the weight shifts to the target-side foot.

On the downswing, you can think of your weight increasingly being transferred to your left side as the club is coming down. Your upper body will move to the left. Your head should stay as close to its starting point as possible, with your shoulders rotating around your head as if your head were the hub of a wheel.

A common mistake of people with little athletic aptitude or training is to start to swing the club from the top of the swing. You must start with the legs; the arms will follow at the proper time. The mistake of "hitting from the top" is similar to one often made by people who don't know how to throw a baseball. They often start with the right leg, then throw with the right arm, whereas the athlete starts with the left-leg step, then throws, then the right leg follows.

Once the golf swing is started from the legs, the hips and shoulders will follow naturally. All you have to do is guide your leading arm (left) through the ball. Your follow-through will turn your body with the shot. Your hands will finish high. And as you finish, your belt buckle should be aimed at the target.

Instead of trying to "hit" the ball, which may lead to mental and physical errors, just think of pulling the clubhead *through* the ball with your left arm. Your stroke will be smooth and have a better chance of success with this approach.

The downswing

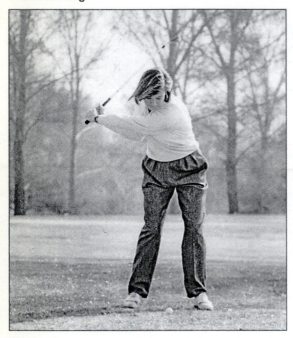

The downswing starts with the legs and a weight shift

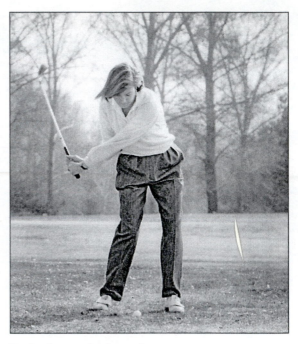

The head moves slightly to right

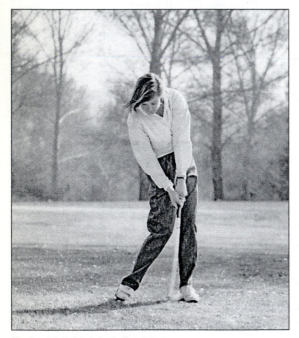

The head is behind the ball at impact

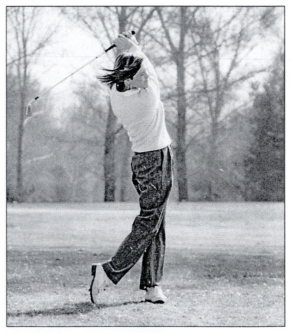

Finish high with belt buckle at target

Checklist for Your Swing

1. "Turn" the club back from the ball by turning your hips and shoulders. Don't "pick up" the club.
2. Make the left arm a lever when you sweep the club back on your backswing. Don't bend your left arm at the elbow.
3. Keep your head centered as the hub of your swing.
4. Turn your left shoulder under your chin.
5. Break your wrists at the top of your backswing.
6. The club should be parallel or nearly parallel to the ground at the top of the backswing.
7. Start the club downward with your left hip.
8. After your hips and shoulders have turned, your arms should swing past your head.
9. Your weight should have shifted from the inside of your right foot to the ball of your left foot, and your belt buckle should be pointing toward the target.
10. The club should swing from the inside out.
11. Finish with your hands high.

Point of Aim

Most people just walk up to the ball, position the body in a way they think will get the ball to the target, then swing. Others are a little more precise. They set their feet, then lay down a club so that it is touching both sets of toes, and look to see if their feet are aligned with the target. These are not the best methods, however. In fact, if you hit the ball straight, it will likely go to the right of where you intended it to go.

Instead, to aim the shot, stand about eight feet behind the ball and visualize an imaginary line to your target. Then step to the side and set your feet—keeping that imaginary line in view. Now swing. Your shot will be more accurate this way.

Aim at a spot on the back of the ball. On a wood shot, your swing will bring the clubhead gently across the grass as it "sweeps" through the ball. On an iron shot, you should hit down and under the ball. If you are hitting down properly with an iron, you will take a divot of grass after you have hit the shot.

If the ball didn't go where you wanted it, ask yourself what was wrong. Was it foot placement? Was it a loose grip, which allowed the club to slip in your hand at impact? Check your foot placement and grip after the shot. If they were off, make a mental note and correct them for the next shot. But don't try to make corrections in your swing while on the course.

Lay a club along your stance to check your aim

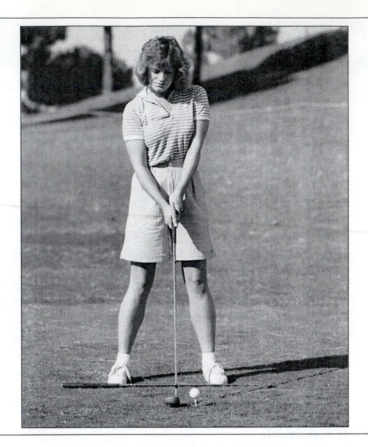

Often it is foot placement that throws off your aim. If the ball went in a different direction than you intended, just place your club on the ground touching both of your toes. Now step back and see where the line of the club is pointing. If the ball went in the direction of the club rather than where you thought it would go, then begin checking your foot alignment before each shot. This simple technique has straightened out many poorly aligned shots. You should use this technique often on the practice tee.

Remember that the ball always goes where you hit it! It may not go where you want it to go, but it goes where you hit it and how you hit it. If it drifts right (a *fade* or a *slice*) or left (a *draw* or a *hook*), you caused it. If it flies out straight and true for 250 yards, you did it. So there is no sense getting angry with your club or the ball. You did it. That's why you should be able to forget the bad shot without getting upset. No one has ever played a perfect golf round. Some people are just a little more consistent than others. To become a better golfer, you just have to make improvements in your consistency. Don't ever count on being perfect. Being perfect is only for saints, not for golfers.

Imparting Spin to the Ball

The basic movement of the golf swing is not very difficult. What causes so many problems is the spin of the ball. Most people hit to the right. To correct this, they aim to the left, but this induces a slice spin. What they need to do is to swing to the right, then the ball will go to the left.

To illustrate how spin is imparted to the ball, imagine you have a water glass on the table and you want it to spin clockwise or counterclockwise—how would you hit it? You would slap the glass with the palm of your right hand, drawing your hand across it. Likewise, to hit a ball that will spin clockwise and drift to the right (a fade or a slice), you do exactly the same, because you can control the face of the golf club with the palm of your right hand (if your hand is placed on the club properly).

Imparting spin to the ball on purpose is something that the pros often do. As a beginner, you should hit straight. Once you have mastered that, you can start to spin the ball.

Choice of Club and Your Swing

You should know how far you hit each club, so choose the club that can do the job for you without your swinging extra hard. In fact, if there is any doubt in your mind, take a little more (longer) club and swing easier. That is, if you are

How spin is imparted to a ball

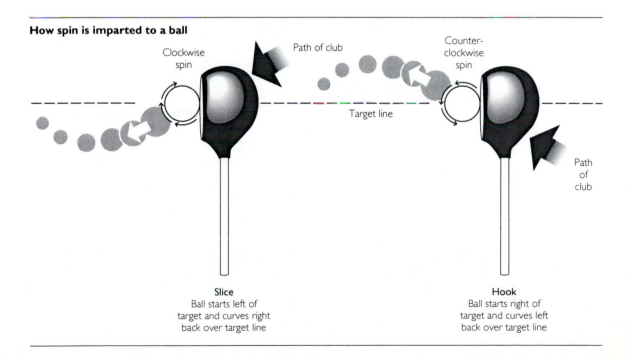

Slice
Ball starts left of
target and curves right
back over target line

Hook
Ball starts right of
target and curves left
back over target line

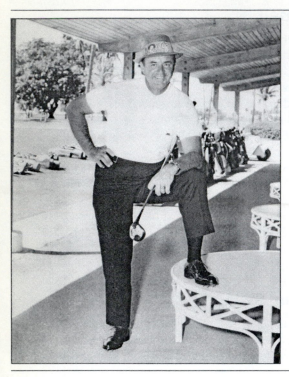

Sam Says:

"I always use the key to move the club back to the address position. I like to pull down with the left hand. The left shoulder shouldn't leave the target line. It works along that line."

not sure whether you should use a 4-iron or a 5-iron, take the 4-iron and swing easier. Don't take the 5-iron and swing harder.

Keys for Your Swing

Every pro and amateur uses certain keys to guide the swing. One key may be to pull down with the left hand, another might be to pull down with the right hand, or to tuck the elbow in on the downswing, or to swing to the right pocket. Still another might be to turn the right knee toward the ball, or turn the hips to the green.

Try several keys to tune yourself into your swing. Use whatever key works. You may even find that the key that works this year doesn't work next year. We haven't yet found a skeleton key that works for all golfers.

Once you make your commitment from the top if the swing, there is no chance for recovery. If you try to correct it on the way down, you are in trouble. So find the key that will get you through your swing the most consistently.

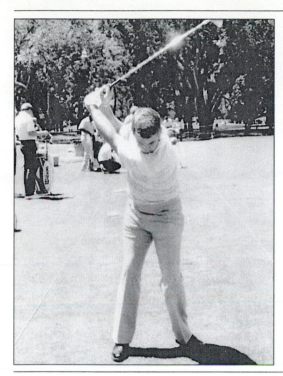

J.C. Says:

"I turn my shoulders toward the ball, leading with the left shoulder. Sometimes I lead with my right shoulder, and sometimes I try to move in front of the ball with the top of my body, but the left shoulder is my major key. I take the club back with the left shoulder and start down with it. Shoulders and hips should be level. The only reason that your right shoulder is lower than your left is because your right hand is lower on the club. I don't use a whole lot of hand action through the ball. I think that people who are "handsy" hit the ball a lot higher."

Summary

1. Your grip should have the back of your left hand and the palm of your right facing the target. The pressure should be felt in the palm of your left hand and the fingers of your right.

2. Your stance should have your feet about shoulder width apart, with your knees slightly flexed and bent inward.

3. Your backswing should be low and toward the inside, with your lead shoulder in control.

4. Your downswing should start with your legs moving forward. Your hips and shoulders will follow without your thinking about them. You need to think only of controlling the club by guiding it downward and through the ball with your left arm.

5. Always swing easy. Let the club do the work. If you need more distance, use a longer club.

6. Remember: Have a firm grip, keep your head down, and swing easy.

5

Making Corrections in Your Swing

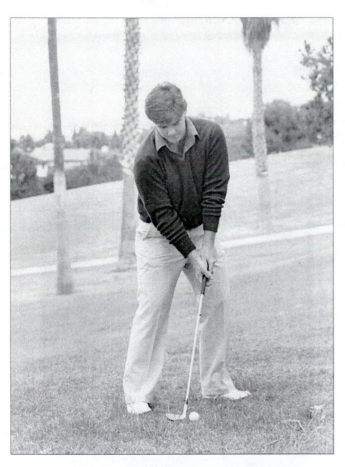

Outline

f your swing is not doing what you want it to do, you may need to make some adjustments. They should be made on the practice tee, not on the course.

Slicing

Slicing (imparting a spin to the ball that makes it go right for right-handers) can usually be corrected by one or more of the following adjustments:

- *If you are hitting the ball with the clubface open*—do not allow the clubface to open during your backswing, or concentrate on releasing your wrists with a counterclockwise action during the downswing, or move your hands a bit farther to the right on your grip.

- *If your upper body is moving past the ball before the clubhead gets to it*—start your swing with your knees, and keep your head behind the ball until after impact.

- *If you are hitting across the ball from the outside in*—start your backswing with your elbow tucked in, concentrate on starting your downswing with your legs, and use a low inside sweep of the club.

Main causes of slicing

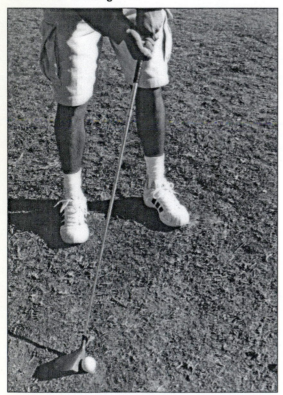

Open face at impact

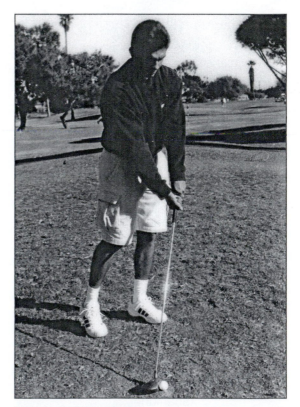

Body ahead of ball at impact

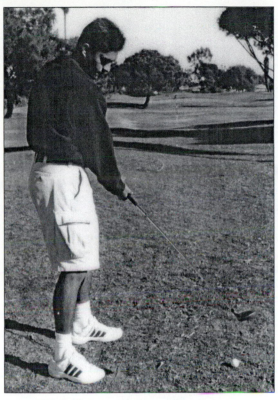

Cutting the ball: Swing path of outside-in

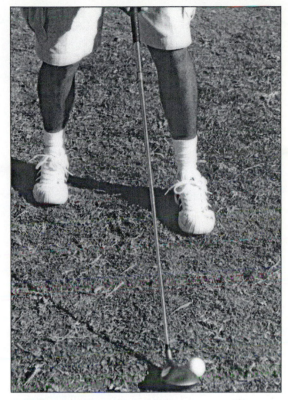

Solution: Relax forearms and close stance

✓	*Checklist for Slicing*

1. Is your stance open (target-side foot farther away from the ball than the other foot)?
2. Is your lower hand (right hand for right-handers) too strong?
3. Are you standing too close to the ball?
4. Is your swing too upright (that is, are you taking it straight up from the ball)?
5. Are you swinging from the outside in?

The slice versus the hook

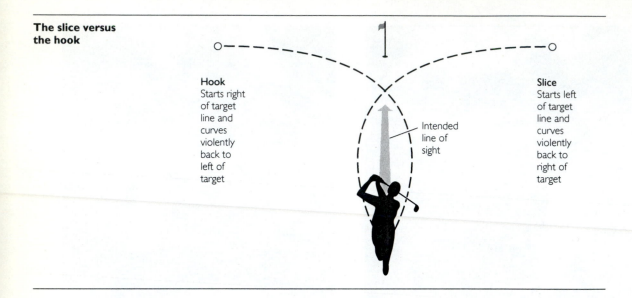

Hook
Starts right of target line and curves violently back to left of target

Intended line of sight

Slice
Starts left of target line and curves violently back to right of target

- Check to see that your forearms are relaxed. If they are not relaxed, they will not allow your wrists to roll enough when you are contacting the ball, so your clubface will be open at impact.
- Close your stance a bit (left foot forward).

Hooking

Hooking (imparting a spin on the ball that makes it curve left for a right-hander) is usually caused by a closed clubface (facing to the left of the desired line of flight). It can be adjusted by:

- Moving your hands a little to the left in your grip.
- Starting your backswing with your left hand firmly in control. It should stay in control through the downswing also.
- Checking your right wrist at the top of your backswing to see if it is under the club as it should be. If it is to the side, it indicates that your wrists are too sloppy and are probably working too much at contact. You want to reduce wrist action throughout the swing.
- Starting your downswing with your legs by shifting your weight toward the target.

Main causes of hooking

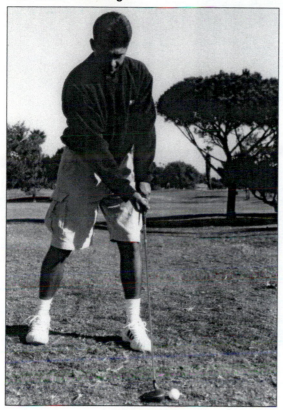

Hitting ball with closed face

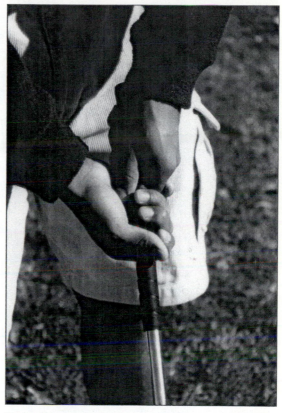

Too strong a grip and overactive hands

 Checklist for Correcting a Hook

1. Is your stance closed (target-side foot farther forward than your other foot)?
2. Is your top hand (left hand for right-handers) too strong?
3. Are you standing too far from the ball?
4. Is your swing too flat (that is, are you taking it around your body rather than upward)?
5. Are you overemphasizing the inside-out aspect of your swing?

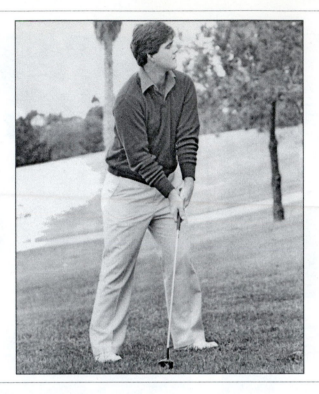

Topping the Ball

Topping the ball (hitting too high on the ball) is a common error that can be corrected by:

- Setting up closer to the ball with less body bend. If you are too crouched in your stance, you probably straighten out as you swing down. So start with a more upright stance.
- Set up with the ball farther back in your stance so that you will hit it sooner.
- Be sure that your right knee stays bent. Straightening it on the backswing will tend to keep your shoulders too high during the downswing. This will result in topping the ball.
- Keep your head in one spot during your swing. If your head raises up, you will probably top the ball.
- Just swing smoothly. Swinging too hard will tend to make you raise your body and head.
- Keep your wrists cocked longer on the downswing.
- Concentrate on pulling the club down with your left arm.

Shanking is caused by hitting too close to the shaft

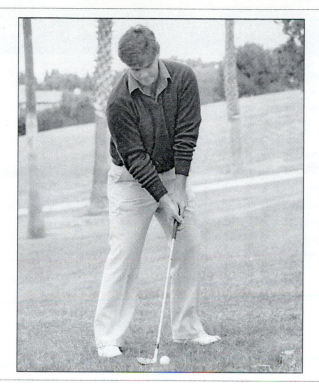

Shanking

Shanking (hitting the ball too close to the shaft of the club) is caused by swinging too wide and hitting with the shaft of the club rather than the clubface. These tips may help:

- Relax your hands and arms. You have been trying too hard.
- Be sure that your grip pressure stays the same throughout your swing.
- Keep your right elbow close to your body and swing inside to outside.

Scuffing

Scuffing (hitting behind the ball) can often be remedied by:

- Keeping a firm base, not sagging on your right side or bending your right knee too much.
- Making sure that your weight shifts from your left side during the backswing.
- Making sure your weight shifts fully by moving your legs early to get your weight forward before you make contact with the ball.
- Keeping your wrists cocked longer.

> ### ✓ *Checklist for a Problem-Free Swing*
>
> 1. Start the club back low and to the inside with a turn of your hips and shoulders while keeping your target-side arm straight.
> 2. Keep your head over the ball, and think of your head as the center of the hub of your swing.
> 3. Turn your target-side shoulder under your head as you reach the top of your backswing.
> 4. Your wrists should be relaxed and "break" at the top of your backswing. This should bring your club approximately parallel with the ground.
> 5. Start the club downward with a forward push from your rear leg, then a turn of your hips, then your shoulders.
> 6. Visualize the clubhead as the end of a rope that you are swinging with your shoulder and target arm. Think of your arm and club as the rope. Your swing should feel that you are swinging the rope from the inside to the outside—from close to your body outward toward the ball. Stay relaxed, and your wrists will release naturally.
> 7. As you finish your swing, your weight will be on your target foot, your hips will be facing the target, and your hands will be high as they finish the swing.

Skying

Skying (hitting too high) can be corrected by:

- Taking a square or slightly closed stance.
- Teeing the ball higher but moving it back in your stance.
- Making certain that you get a full backswing. Don't rush it.
- Sweeping the ball rather than hitting down at it.

General Comments on Correcting Your Swing

Remember that golf is a game of opposites. Swing to the right if you want the ball to go left. Swing to the left if you want the ball to go right. Also, a good golf swing requires the utmost in concentration and coordination. Finally, proper practice is essential.

Summary

1. Because the golf swing requires a very fine coordination, many errors can affect it.

2. Slicing the ball (imparting a spin that makes the ball curve right for right-handers) occurs because the clubface is open when it contacts the ball. This can be corrected by:
   - Closing the stance
   - Swinging from the inside out
   - Keeping your head behind the ball at impact

3. Hooking the ball (a spin that makes the ball go left for right-handers) occurs because the clubface is closed at impact. It can usually be corrected by:
   - Starting the downswing with a proper weight shift
   - Changing the grip
   - Keeping the left hand firmly in control

4. Topping the ball (hitting too high on the ball) can usually be corrected by one or more of the following:
   - Setting up closer to the ball
   - Setting the ball farther back in your stance
   - Keeping your head down during the swing

5. Shanking the ball (hitting the ball too close to the shaft of the club) is caused by swinging too wide. It can usually be corrected by keeping the right elbow close to the body or by relaxing more during the swing.

6. Scuffing (hitting behind the ball) can be corrected by getting a proper weight shift or keeping the wrists cocked longer.

7. Skying (hitting too high) can be corrected by:
   - Closing the stance
   - Teeing the ball lower
   - Relaxing more during the swing
   - Sweeping the ball rather than hitting down on it

6 *Expecting the Unexpected*

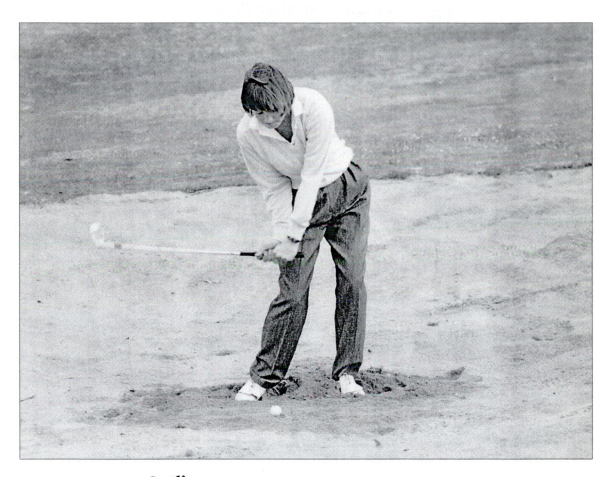

Outline

Ben Hogan said that if you hit five good shots a round, you have probably played as well as you can. When it comes to golf, you can't avoid getting into trouble time after time on the golf course.

It has often been said that golf is a series of recovery shots. Since the ball almost never goes exactly where you want it to go, you must always expect the unexpected. Here is some help on playing the less than ideal shots.

Playing Shots from Nonflat Lies

Downhill Lies

If the ball is on a slope that is heading down in the direction you are hitting, it is called a *downhill lie*. Take a practice swing to find the point where the clubhead will touch the turf. It should be towards your uphill foot. Now take your stance with the ball back toward your uphill foot (right foot for right-handers). This will put the ball closer to the lowest point of your swing. Choose a club with more loft than you would usually play from that distance. This is because the slope of the ground changes the amount of loft you will need for a proper shot. Aim left of the target. Use a more upright arm swing and less body rotation on this shot—and stay down!

Downhill lie: The ball moves backward in your stance

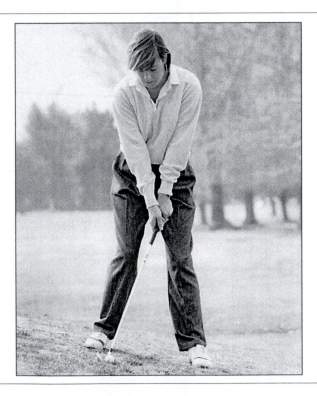

Uphill lie: The ball moves forward in your stance

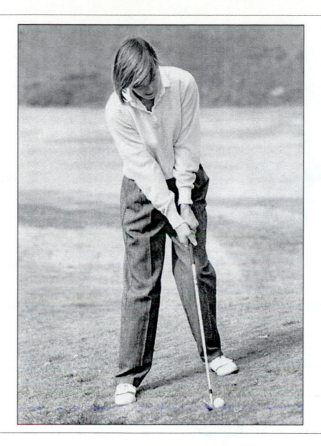

Uphill Lies

Hitting *uphill* requires the opposite approach. Take a practice swing to find the point where the clubhead will touch the ground. Your stance will then have the ball closer to your uphill foot (left foot for right-handers). Take a club with less loft, because the angle of the ground gives you the effect of more loft. Keep more weight on the downhill leg. Aim to the right of the target. On this shot, as with the downhill shot, use more arm swing and less body rotation.

Sidehill Lie with the Ball Lower Than Your Feet

Take a lesser club (a higher-numbered club with a shorter shaft), because you will have a longer swing. Hold the club high on the grip. Stand closer than usual to the ball. Bend your knees. Aim more to the left, because the ball will probably fade. And keep your head down and as motionless as possible.

Sidehill lie with ball below feet: Stand more erect and move your grip up on the club

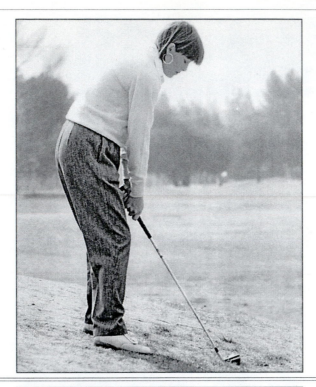

Sidehill lie with ball above feet: Stand more erect and choke up on the club

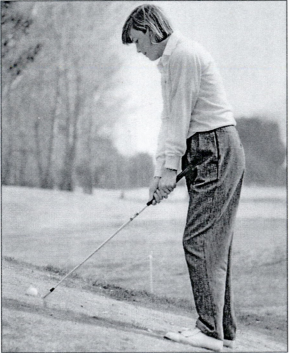

Sidehill Lie with the Ball Higher Than Your Feet

Take a bit more club (a lower-numbered club with a longer shaft), because you will have to choke down on it and will get less than the proper distance from it. Stand more erect than usual, but keep more weight on your heels. Then aim more to the right, because the ball will generally hook.

Getting Out of Trouble

Playing from the Rough

The high grass (the *rough*) is there to make your shot more difficult. And the more grass you hit during the downswing, the more difficult your shot will be to make. So by taking a more upright swing, you will hit less grass.

If you want distance from your iron shot, play it closer to your rear foot, close the clubface a bit, and hit a punch-shot down at the ball. Use a lot of right hand, but don't try to "power" it. The ball should come out low, probably to the left, and should roll a long way after it hits. If you choose to play a wood, open the clubface and hit similarly to your iron shot.

If you want height, play the ball more forward, take a full swing, but use a lot of wrist on the shot. The grass will slow down your full fast swing.

The rough: The tall grass makes solid contact with the ball difficult

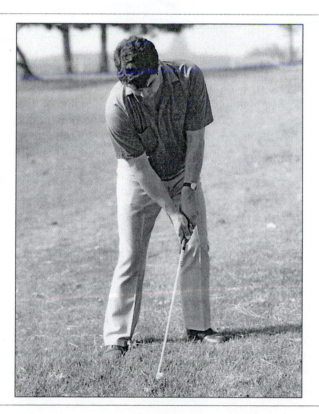

Takes a more upright swing in the rough

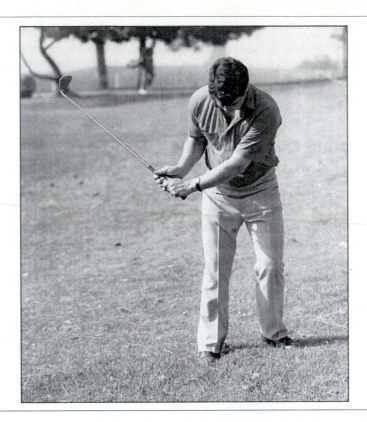

If the grass is growing away from your intended line of flight, it will tend to slow your clubhead, so take one more club (a club one number lower than you would ordinarily use) to overcome the resistance. If the grass is growing toward the intended line of flight, take one less club. The ball will probably go high, but will roll more than normal.

Playing in the Woods

If you have hit your shot into the trees and don't have a clear shot out, don't be afraid to take a 2-iron or 3-iron and hit a short punch-shot back onto the fairway.

If your ball is lying against a tree or other object, use your putter to knock it into a more playable lie. You may even have to hit it left-handed, but that one stroke should improve your lie considerably.

Keep trying in the face of bad luck or disappointment. Face the danger of each stroke, and curb the desire to take chances that are beyond hope. Play within yourself at all times. You probably can't hit the ball through the tree.

Playing from the Fairway Bunker

When you land in a *fairway bunker*, you will want to get distance from your shot, so use a long iron. Use one or two irons more—that is, one or two numbers lower—than you would need to play from the grass. (Go up one iron if the sand is light, two irons if it is heavy.) Some pros will even use a 4-wood on occasion—if the ball is sitting high. But don't hit a wood if there is a chance of hitting the sand first.

First wiggle your feet into the sand until your stance is firm. Play the ball back in your stance so that you are sure to hit it before you hit the sand. Reduce your lower body movement. And, above all, get out of the trap in one shot.

If the ball is lower than your feet, grip the club as high as possible, bend your knees to get down to the ball, and aim left, just as in the typical bunker shot. If the ball is above your feet, just do everything the opposite way. Choke up on the club, stand more erect, and aim to the right, because the ball will tend to fly right from this position.

On a fairway bunker shot, you want to keep your feet and legs as still as possible. Too much movement and weight transfer in a bunker shot will cause the sand to slip a little, and you may hit the ball fat or thin. Try to hit the ball

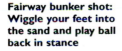

Fairway bunker shot: Wiggle your feet into the sand and play ball back in stance

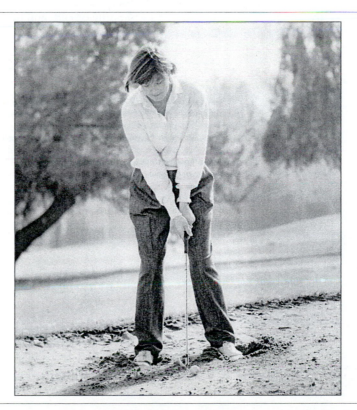

✓ *Checklist for Playing from a Fairway Bunker*

1. Play the ball closer to your rear foot—toward the back of your stance.
2. Make sure that your hands are positioned well ahead of the ball.
3. When you execute your backswing, pick the club up sharply.
4. Drive the club down through the ball after you have completed your backswing.
5. Make sure that you execute the shot by hitting down at the ball with a punch-shot.

very smoothly. Some people hit down on the ball and take sand, and some people like to pick it up off the sand.

Playing from a Divot

A divot is a piece of turf dislodged by a club. Playing from a divot hole requires that the ball be played more off the right foot than usual. If you are using a wood, use a more lofted one than you ordinarily would, and hit down on the ball to make it pop up more quickly.

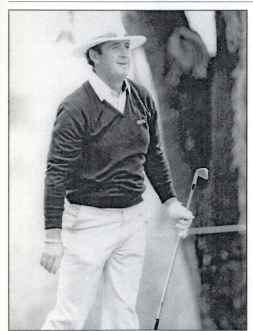

J.C. Says:

"When I was first on the tour I tried to be a hero in the woods. I generally failed. Now I play smarter. Remember, golf is a game of misses, anyway. And your chances of missing are less on the fairway than in the woods.

One time up at Muirfield, on a par 5, my ball went right up against a tree. I had no swing at all. So I took a sand wedge and turned it upside down and hit it left-handed. I must have hit it about 175 yards. Every once in a while you can hit a great shot like that. But you have to practice it. I will hit some left-handed sand wedges on the practice tee every once in a while.

A great shot like that can give you a real lift and charge you up so that you play better."

Playing from the Water

Hitting out of the water is best avoided. Take the penalty, especially if the ball is covered by more than a half inch of water. If you must play it, hit down on it so that you can hit as close to the ball as possible to prevent the water in front of your clubhead from pushing the ball out of the way. Don't touch the water with your club before you hit the ball, or it's another penalty stroke.

Playing in Adverse Weather Conditions

Playing in the Wind

The wind can affect golfers very negatively. It makes them want to hurry when they should be slowing down. A shot on a windy day requires that you think more about what you are going to do.

First, you want to get an idea of how hard and in which direction the wind is blowing. You can lick your finger and stick it in the air to determine a slight breeze, or you can pick up some loose grass and let it drift from your hand to get a better idea of the wind's velocity and direction.

We all know that wind can swirl. Also, it may blow harder, or even in a different direction, on different parts of the same fairway. So look up in the trees to see which way the leaves are blowing, and look at the flag on the pin. Is the wind swirling, or is it fairly consistent in its direction?

If the wind is with you, use one, two, or even three more clubs than usual, and keep the ball down a little. You can play the ball more off your left foot. Don't try to hit the ball hard into the wind. Just swing smoothly. The harder you hit the ball, the more backspin you put on it. The combination of the wind and backspin will make the ball go up in the air and get caught in more wind. Choke down on your club a little and hit the ball easy. Let the wind be your friend.

If the wind is against you, take about one more club for each 10 miles per hour that the wind is blowing. Play your shot off your right foot.

In hitting a driver into the wind, tee it down a little. Choke down on the club and keep your weight more on your left side and keep your shoulders more level. If anything, feel like your left shoulder is a little lower than your right. That will definitely make you hit the ball lower.

To hit it high, do just the opposite. Set up with the ball a little forward in your stance, drop your right shoulder, and set up a little on your right side. If you do this, the ball will definitely come up in the air.

If you are playing into a cross wind, where will you have to aim to get the ball where you want it? Look at the trees near your target to get an idea of what the wind is doing. Use one more club than usual.

The wind generally blows harder and more consistently higher up, so your more lofted clubs may be more greatly affected than your lower-numbered clubs. Once you choose your club, make certain that you relax your swing. Don't hurry it, and don't hit harder. The increased backspin on a harder hit may make the ball go much higher than you want. Nature has provided enough variables to your game—don't add any more.

If the wind is blowing right to left, just hit your ball out to the right a little bit. Never try to curve the ball with the wind unless you are hitting a tee shot or a very long shot and you want to ride the wind to get the maximum distance out of the shot. If you are hitting the ball well, you might do as we do and work the ball against the wind. Then when it hits on the green, it will stop right there.

If you're working the ball downwind, or if you are turning the ball, you could be in trouble. For example, if you have a right-to-left wind and you hit a little hook, once the wind turns it to the left and gets behind it, the ball won't stop until it has gone a couple of fairways to your left.

Playing in the Rain

The rain often has a greater psychological effect than the wind. One is tempted to either stay in the clubhouse or to hurry the game up and hit the clubhouse for cup of coffee and a bout of hero stories. But that's not the way to approach it. Remember that when the devil invented this game, he decided to pit all the forces of nature against us. So take up the challenge!

The first thing to remember is to settle into a firm solid stance. You might have to clean your spikes before every shot. You definitely don't want to slip, so clean your cleats with a tee or a green-repair tool, and you will have eliminated one variable.

Eliminate as many variables as you can. Hit every shot straight. If you try to fade or draw, the rain will probably slow or stop the spin, and your shot won't come back the way you had planned.

Don't try for extra distance to compensate for the soggy grass. Just hit the ball (instead of the grass) first, so that the wet grass doesn't get between the clubface and the ball. Don't try to break par, but instead settle for a consistent game. You are generally better off using one more club than normal but taking a shorter backswing.

Remember that you can drop away from *casual water* (water that is not part of the original course design) on the fairway and that you can move the ball on the green if there is casual water between you and the hole. No sense causing yourself more problems than you need.

Developing the Right Attitude

Your attitude toward bad lies is critical. If you let these essentials of the golf game ruin your attitude, disrupt your next shot, or take the fun out of the game, you don't understand golf. It is a game of the unexpected.

It is the challenge of these so-called "bad breaks" that makes the game so great. They are the situations that stimulate our intellects and test our talents. Remember that only the current shot is important. The last shot has been played. And good or bad, it must be forgotten.

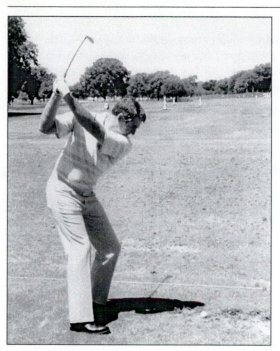

J.C. Says:

"Sam was always a master at working the ball against the wind. There's nothing prettier than watching a man take a 5-iron and hit a little fade into the wind just enough to hold it straight. It fights the wind all the way, then when it gets over the green it drops like a snowflake.

The fairway bunker shot has always been one of the hardest shots in the game for me. If the ball is sitting fairly clean, then I can usually handle it. But if the ball is sitting down a little bit, I find it a very difficult shot for me always—it doesn't matter how well I'm playing."

People who can't handle the hills and dales, the traps and water, the high grass and the trees should invent another game played on flat Astro-turf in which there are no bad lies. And they could yell "bore" on their errant shots.

Accept the challenge of the game and realize that you will never play a perfect round in 18 strokes. The "bogeyman" (in the form of traps and trees and so forth) lies in wait at every turn

Confidence is essential in making recovery shots. For this reason, don't try to make a "career" shot when the odds are against it. That little voice inside you may be saying "I think I can," but what odds would a professional odds-maker give you?

You may want to opt for hooking around a clump of trees and landing on the green. But what are the odds? The optimist in you, thinking of what might be, should give in to the realist in you, who knows what you can do.

In planning for your best shot, you must take into account the potential problems—the out-of-bounds, the water, the traps. Then select the proper club and the best target area. Next, you must clearly "see" the shot you are going to make. Ignore the obstacles—the out-of-bounds, the pond, the bunkers—because you already considered them in your shot selection. Now it is time to focus all your attention on the positive.

The worse the conditions or the lies are, the more conservatively you must play. Save your hero shots for the days when the conditions are perfect and your lies are flat.

Summary

1. Golf courses are purposely designed to make things difficult for you—with bunkers, woods, and rough. Nature often frustrates you as well with wind and rain. These are the factors that make golf the challenging game it is.

2. Golf has been described as a series of recovery shots.

3. The worse the conditions or the lie, the more conservatively you must play.

4. Save your hero shots for the days when the conditions are perfect and your lies are flat.

7   *Near the Green*

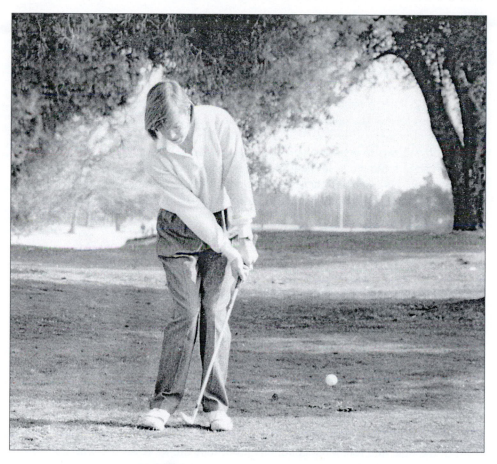

Outline

Most of your shots will be made from close to the green. It is the approach shots, the chipping, pitching, and putting, that test the true skills of the golfer. A National Golf Foundation survey found that 56 percent of all golf shots take place around the green (13 percent chips and 43 percent putts). When you contrast those percentages with the 25 percent wood shots, 14 percent iron shots, and 5 percent classified as "trouble shots," you can see the immense importance of being effective around the greens.

From 150 yards out, you are in scoring area. This is the area in which you must use effective strategy and a technically effective swing in order to score well.

Sizing Up Your Approach Shot

Check the marker bushes to see about how far away from the hole you are. (Most courses have a bush on each side of the fairway 150 yards from the green.) Then look at the pin placement. Is it far away? Is it close? What is the slope of the green?

Your objective is to get on the green, not necessarily to sink your 150-yard approach shot. If the pin is set near the fringe, plan on playing it safe. If the pin is set deep on the green and there is a trap behind the green, play it safe to the middle of the green. If the pin is near the front edge and is protected by traps, play it safe in the middle. If the green slopes and you can hit downhill from the pin, do that. Remember, it is better to be safe than sorry.

From 150 yards out we might hit a little 7-iron or a full 8. But if there is a lot of trouble in front of the green or the shot has to carry over water we might hit a full 7 or an easy 6. You never want to use a club that requires you to hit it absolutely perfectly to get to the hole.

Weigh all these options and decide on your strategy. Pull out the club that will do the job. Mentally picture your shot. Take a practice swing that duplicates your mental picture. Settle into your stance, address the ball, and swing easy.

Pitching and Chipping

The *pitch* is a high shot that will stop close to where it landed. The *chip* will hit short of the hole and roll. Most golfers feel that they are more secure with the ball rolling than flying—so if you are close to the green, the chip shot is generally preferred.

Some people like to swing with little or no break in their wrists. They use the Y-shape of the arms and club shaft and keep the Y inflexible. Other people choose to hit primarily with their wrists. We prefer the straighter-arm type of shot.

The important thing is that you want your weight on your left side, but you want a little transfer of weight—even if it is just from the inside to the outside of your left leg. It doesn't have to shift completely to your right leg. Stay on your left side and play it with your left arm.

It is in the pitching and chipping that touch becomes essential. Depending on the distance from your target area, you will have to adjust your backswing. Use less backswing for the short shots and more for the longer ones. These are the shots you can practice in your backyard or in a park.

The Pitch Shot

The pitch shot is generally done with a 9-iron or a pitching wedge. Your stance should be narrow but open to the green. The club should move rather slowly, with just enough speed to get the ball where you want it. The slower speed will help achieve good height on the ball.

The Chip Shot

The chip shot can be done with any club, depending on how much you want the ball to carry in flight and how far you want it to roll. You can also control the amount of flight and roll by where you place the ball. If it is placed farther forward in your stance, it will fly higher; if farther back, it will go lower but roll more.

On chip shots, use a less-lofted club. With your weight on the left side and your feet close together, open up the stance with your feet and shoulders until you feel like you're almost going to putt the ball. Use the same type of stroke that you do when putting.

For a little pitch shot, you may want to choke down on the grip a little, then just open the blade with your hands. You don't open the blade, then take your grip. Take your grip, then twist your wrists just a little. Twist it open with your left hand and maintain that angle.

Keep your weight on the left side. Bend your knees as you sit down to the ball. Point the end of the club grip at your left hip. This will put your hands ahead of the ball, which is of primary importance in chipping.

With your head as motionless as possible, swing your Y-shape pendulum (arms and club) from your shoulders. Your hands must stay ahead of the ball throughout the entire swing so that you will be hitting down on the ball. Let your left arm firmly control this shot.

Take a short, compact backswing, turning the blade over a little bit as you strike the ball. Always hit down on it; never think of swinging up. And keep your hands slightly ahead of the ball at impact. You will slide the clubface just under the ball with your hand as you hit it. The ball will come off very softly and pop up.

On a little chip-and-run, you can land the ball on the fringe, but it is better on the green. Use whatever lofted club you need to make it hit the green and roll to the hole. If your lie is right on the fringe, you might be able to take a 4-, 5-, or 6-iron and stand just as you do when you putt.

The chip shot

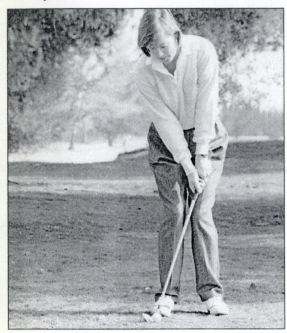

Stance for chip: Ball back in stance

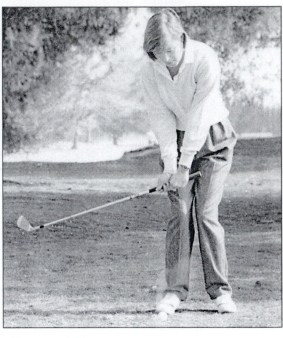

Swing the Y-pendulum

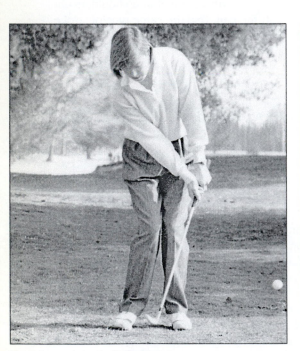

Hands firm and ahead of ball at impact

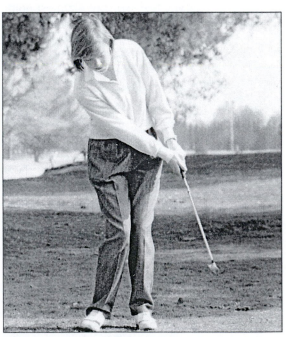

Maintain firm wrists in follow-through

Expected ratios of ball in-the-air to roll for pitching wedge, 9, and 7

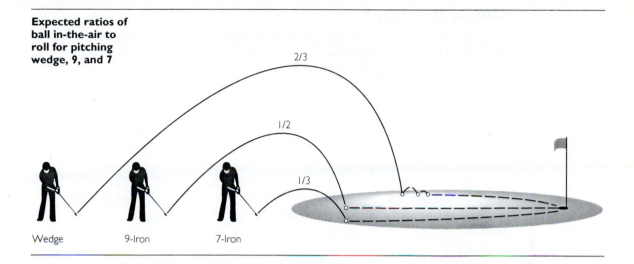

In chipping, many players like to aim for a spot about 5 feet in from the fringe. The choice of club will give you a good idea as to how far the ball will roll after it hits. Here are the expected ratios of ball-in-the-air to the roll for three clubs:

- Pitching wedge: two-thirds of the distance in the air and one-third roll
- 9-iron: half the distance in the air and half roll
- 7-iron: one-third of the distance in the air and two-thirds roll

If you are playing with a tailwind, use the chip-and-run rather than the high chip shot to keep the ball on the ground longer.

✓ *Checklist for the Chip Shot*

1. Hit down on the ball, and do not attempt to scoop it up.
2. Use an open stance (that is, your target-side foot is away from the line of flight).
3. Keep your hands ahead of the ball at the address.
4. Execute the chip shot with the arms and shoulders—no body motion.
5. Pick a spot on the green as a target for your ball to hit, and allow the ball to roll to the hole. Your ball should be in the air as little as possible and should roll as long as possible.
6. Your target area should be an imaginary 3-foot circle surrounding the hole.

Out of the Traps

So your ball has landed in a sand trap near the green. Not to worry. Several other golfers have found themselves in a bunker at one time or another. And remember that golf is just a series of recovery shots. So here are a few ways to recover from a trap.

A basic premise on the golf course is that you must get out of the trap on your first shot. Don't try to be a hero and hit the ball over a high overhanging lip if you are not 100 percent certain that you can do it. Play it safe!

The rules state that you can't touch any part of the trap with your club, and you can't move anything in the bunker. You must play the ball as you find it—even if it is in a deep footprint of some inconsiderate oaf playing ahead of you. You are, however, allowed to remove enough debris (sand, leaves, etc.) so that you can see the top of the ball—proof that the rule makers of golf are not as heartless as they sometimes seem.

To get out of the sand, you won't even have to hit the ball. Just hit the sand behind the ball, and the ball will pop out. It is a relatively simple shot.

If your ball is partially buried, use the club with the greatest loft. A sand wedge is the obvious first choice, especially if the ball is fairly high in the sand. If you don't carry a sand wedge, use your pitching wedge. No pitching wedge? Get out your 9-iron. (The pitching wedge or 9-iron might be your first choice for a ball set deeper in the sand, because they will cut deeper than the sand wedge.) If you are not carrying one of these clubs, take out your tennis racket, because you not prepared for a golf game!

Address the Ball

Play the ball off your left heel. Settle your feet into the sand so that you have a firm foothold. Make a note as to the texture of the sand as you wiggle your feet. Is it heavy and course? Is it light and fine? The answer helps determine the amount of power you should impart to your swing. If the sand is softer or lighter, you will need to swing harder. If the sand is hard, your club will not go as deep, so you will not need as much power.

How Hard to Swing

You must decide how much power you will need to get the ball from the sand to your target. You can either vary the speed of your swing or "take" more or less sand. It is easier for most people to keep the same swing and vary the amount of sand they take with the shot. The more sand you take, the less power will be transmitted to the ball. In either case, you will generally have to swing about twice as hard at a ball in the sand as you would at one on the grass to get it to go the same distance.

Another factor to consider in deciding how much sand to take is how you want the ball to react after it hits the ground. The farther back you hit behind the ball, the less backspin you will impart, so the more the ball will "run" after it lands.

Stance and Swing

Take an open stance. Choke down on the grip enough to compensate for the depth of your feet in the sand. (Your shoulders will be closer to the ball because your feet are partially buried.) Adjust your grip so that the clubface is slightly open—the toe (end) of the club farther back than the heel of the club. (The closer you are to the target, the more the clubface will be open.) Aim slightly to the left of your target, because the open clubface will give your shot a slicing effect.

Be careful not to touch the sand or you will lose two strokes. Be sure that your hands are "out in front." This is because you will want to hit down into the sand behind the ball.

Take the club back, and break your wrists early. This will allow you to hit down into the sand. Bring the club back to the outside. Your open stance will

The bunker shot

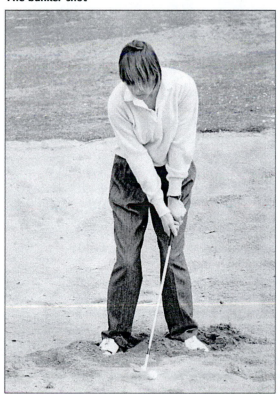

Play ball forward in stance

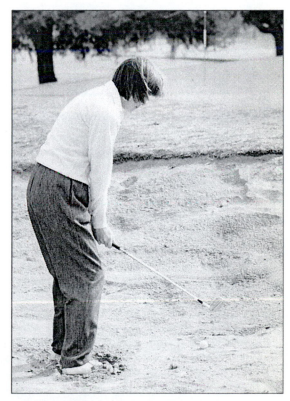

Take more upright, outside-in swing

The bunker shot—continued

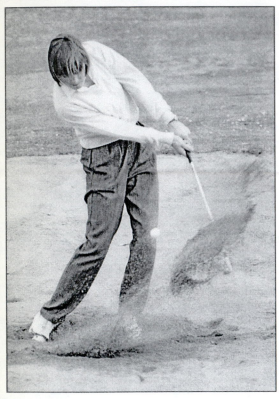

Hit behind the ball

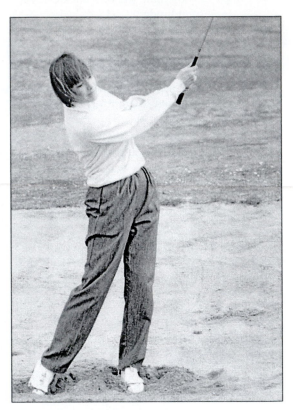

A full follow-through is crucial

make this easier. Take a full smooth swing from the outside in—keeping the clubface slightly open. Contact the sand an inch or two behind the ball. The wide flange of the sand wedge will not allow the clubface to go as deep as the clubs with a narrower lower edge, or flange. So your choice of club will determine how far behind the ball you will aim.

Keep your head down and hit the ball solidly. Then take a full follow-through shifting your weight to your left side. But your whole swing should be done more slowly than your normal tempo. Just relax and don't rush it.

A common error is to try to scoop the ball out of the sand. Instead, you should "blast" it out! The flange of the club will keep the club from going too deep into the sand. Many players find it helpful to think of the ball as if it were sitting right in the middle of a "sand divot." Instead of hitting the ball, then taking the divot, as you would on grass, take a 5- to 6-inch sand divot—making certain that the ball is just a bit behind the middle of the divot you are taking.

If the ball is buried, square or close your clubface. And with a firm grip with the left hand, hit down sharply about an inch behind the ball.

Checklist for Playing a Bunker Shot

1. Visualize your shot with the sand moving the ball. The club should never touch the ball.

2. Make sure that you use a sand wedge.

3. Use an open stance when you address the ball. (Your target-side foot should be farther from the line of flight of the ball, and it should be turned out more than in a fairway shot.)

4. Keep at least 80 percent of your weight on your target-side foot.

5. Do not touch the sand before you make your swing, or it will cost you a two-stroke penalty.

6. As you address the ball, make sure that your hands are behind the ball.

7. Square the clubface with the target, and visualize the club sliding under the ball.

8. Take a full, effortless swing, and hit through the sand, finishing with your hands high.

9. Aim for the largest part of the green (the fat side). Do not try to sink the ball in to the hold from a bunker shot.

10. Maintain confidence that you can execute the shot with the sand moving the ball.

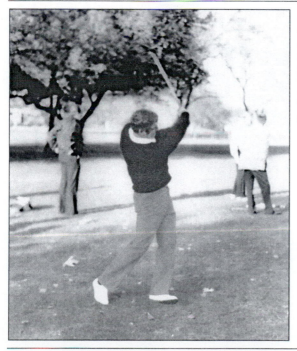

J.C. Says:

"Amateurs usually only see the front of the green. They never seem to look to see where the pin is—it could be 30 yards farther. But it seems that most people with over a 5 handicap just plan to bounce the ball off the front of the green no matter where the pin is. We play in pro-ams every week—and everybody does it. Now with these new courses, with bunkers right in front of the green, you're likely to be in the bunker on your approach shot rather than on the green."

Summary

1. The closer you are to the hole, the more accurate you must be in both distance and aim.
2. The pitch shot, usually made with a pitching wedge or 9-iron, is designed to arc high and stop near the hole.
3. The chip shot is designed to hit near the edge of the green, then roll to the cup.
4. Both pitch and chip shots are made from an open stance with the head held motionless.
5. On shots from traps, you are not allowed to touch the sand with a club except during the shot.

8 *Putting*

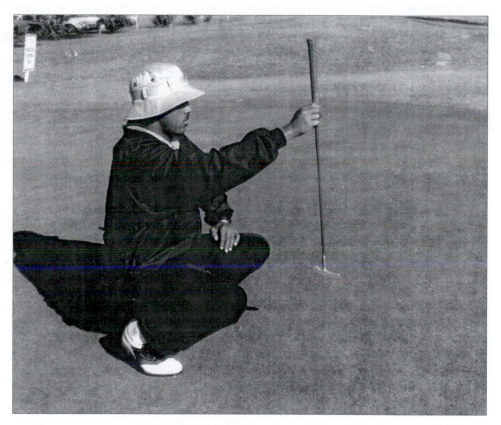

Outline

I t has been said that golf is an athletic game from the tee to the green. After that, it becomes a chess game. Putting is more mental than physical. Every golfer has the strength to putt the ball. What is needed is confidence, relaxation, and concentration. Confidence will come as you learn to read the greens and develop the touch necessary to control your putting for distance. Relaxation comes in part from that confidence and part from the mental techniques that we have already discussed. Then when you know what you are going to do you must concentrate—just like in any other golf shot.

For professionals about 50 percent of their strokes are putts. For amateurs it may be closer to 30 percent. In either case, you can see that putting is very important to your score.

Selecting a Putter

Selecting a putter is best left until after you have developed what you think will be a comfortable stance and stroke. The length of the shaft should be such that when your hands are comfortably on the grip and with the blade resting on the grass, your eyes should be directly over the ball. If you are tall, you will need a longer shaft than a person of average height. If you are short, just choke down on the grip.

The head of the putter is your second concern. A heavy-headed putter will be better for long putts or on slow greens because you do not have to stroke the ball as hard with it—and the harder you stroke, the more likely you are to make a physical mistake. On the other hand, a lighter-headed putter gives you better distance control on short putts and more touch on faster greens.

The angle of the shaft to the blade is also important. When you are in your "perfect" putting stance with you eyes over the ball and your hands close to your body, the sole of the club should be flat on the ground. If everything else about the putter except the lie is good, your pro can bend the shaft to make it lie right for you.

Searching for the right putter is like trying to find the right mate. If you find one that is compatible with you keep it forever.

Putting Technique

The Grip

The first essential of good solid putting is a good grip. The most common grip is started with the palm of the right hand facing the target and the right thumb directly on top of the club. With the left hand on top, the back of the left hand faces the target with the left thumb on top of the club. Most golfers like to overlap the left index finger over the little finger of the right hand.

Another method, called the *cross-handed grip*, has the left hand lower on the grip than the right hand. With this grip it is nearly impossible to bend the left wrist in the stroke. Many pros are now using this grip. The most important

The two most common putting grips

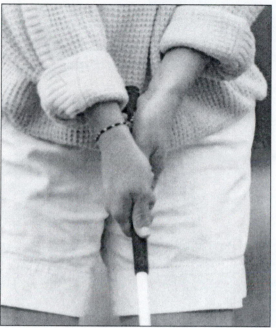

Both thumbs on top of the club and palm facing the target

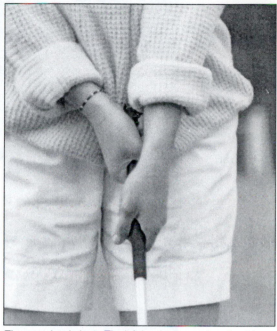

The cross-handed grip: The left hand is lower than the right

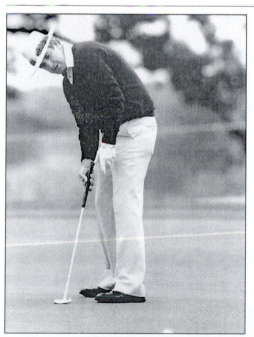

J.C. Says:

"A hot putter on the tour can hide a lot of bad shots. You can't win on the tour if you're a poor putter. But if you're only an average ball striker and a first rate putter, you can win out there."

A third grip option: Palms facing away from your body

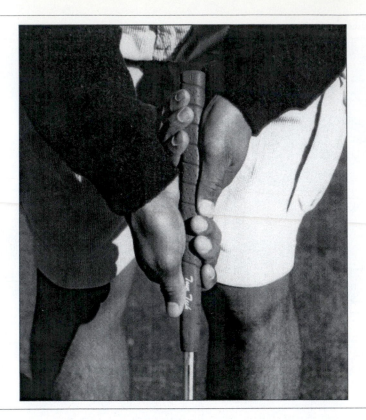

requirement for a good putting grip, however, is that it should allow you to keep the putter head perpendicular to the line of your putt throughout the back-swing and on the follow-through.

If you tend to pull or push your putts, there is still another grip you might want to try. Turn both of your palms away from you, but keep your thumbs on top of the grip. This grip prevents the wrist action that can throw off your putts. Of course, you will have to use the shoulder pendulum stroke.

The grip should be firm but not tight. Tightness will make your hitting muscles tense up, and you want your putting stroke to be smooth and tension free.

The Stance

A solid stance starts with the feet about 12 inches apart. The knees should be slightly bent, with your weight mainly on the left foot. Your head should be over the ball. Probably no technique on the pro tour varies as much as the putting stance. The one constant is that the eyes must be over the ball, and the head should remain motionless.

Normal stance

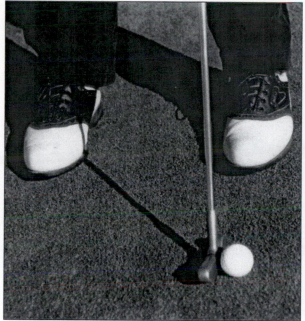

Feet 12 inches apart parallel to target line

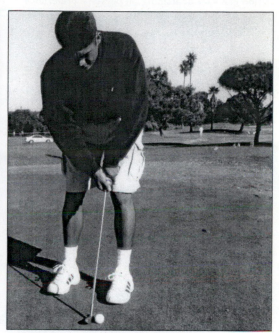

Knees are bent with your eyes over the ball

Many putters keep their toes exactly perpendicular to the line of the putt. This method is used more often by those who putt "from the shoulders." The "wrist putters" often use a slightly open stance.

Ball Alignment

The alignment of the ball should be the same for every putt. A common placement is to have the ball in front of the left foot about one putter blade length in front of the toe. By keeping the ball placement the same on every putt, you can eliminate another variable.

If you have trouble because you break your left wrist before the ball leaves your putter blade, you might place the ball back a few inches closer to the center—perhaps inside your left heel rather than in front of your toes. This will lessen the chances of an early wrist break.

Ball position can vary depending on personal preference

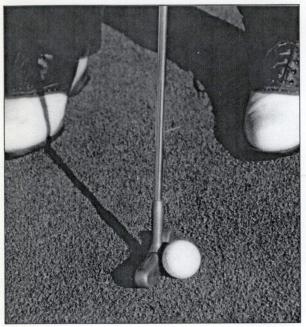

Ball inside left foot

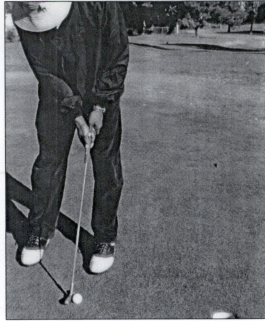

Ball slightly in front of left foot

The Putting Stroke

The putting stroke should be just as grooved as the full swing that you use on your tee shot. The power of the stroke can come from using some combination of wrists, arms, and/or the shoulders. Although most tour players use their wrists and arms primarily, the wrist-action putt can introduce more errors for those who do not have the time to practice daily. Those who use this technique believe that they get a better feel for the long putts, but sacrifice a little on the shorter putts.

For the beginning player, it is generally better to use only shoulder action with no wrist break. To execute this technique, keep your head perfectly still and your eyes directly over the ball. From this position, your arms can swing in a pendulum action from your shoulders around the pivot of your immobile head. By pointing both elbows outward slightly, you will eliminate the possible rotation of the upper arms in the shoulder sockets, which can change the angle of the putter blade and increase the chance of an error. It is very important to meet the center of the ball with the putter blade flat.

Some beginners take the putter too far back, then slow it down as it approaches the ball. Rather, you should accelerate through the ball so that you can control the ball longer on the putter blade. You stroke the ball. You don't punch it.

Some players keep about the same amount of backswing but vary the speed at which they stroke the putter. Most golfers vary the backswing and increase the power of the stroke by taking the club back farther.

Lining Up the Putt

Probably no strategic decision in golf is as complicated as determining how to putt the ball. There are more variables in this shot than any other because the ball is on the ground, and the ground variables outnumber the air variables. The roll of the green, the length of the grass, the grain of the grass, the dampness factor, and the wind all enter into your decision on how to putt.

Before it is your turn, you should be lining up your putt. This way you will save time. Your job on the green is to prepare for your shot, not to be a spectator for others' putts.

In lining up the putt, you should look at it from all sides as you judge the slope of the green and the length and grain of the grass. Start on the low side of the putt trajectory first. Check the break of the green and the grain of the grass. Then walk beyond the hole and check the same things. As you walk back to your ball, pace off the distance from the hole to the ball. This will give you a better idea of how hard to stroke the ball. This is particularly important on long putts.

Line up your putt

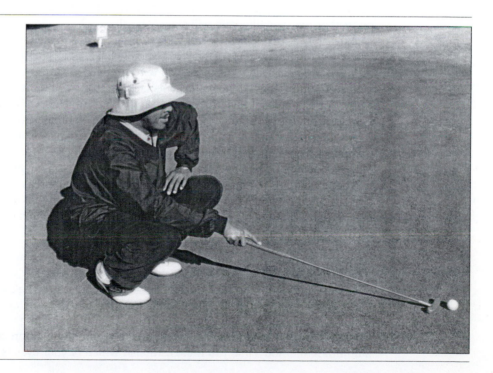

Increase your chances of making a putt

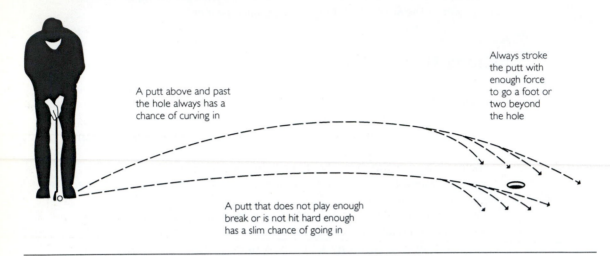

A putt above and past the hole always has a chance of curving in

Always stroke the putt with enough force to go a foot or two beyond the hole

A putt that does not play enough break or is not hit hard enough has a slim chance of going in

Reading the Grain

An essential part of planning your putt is reading the grain. Which way is the shiny side of the grass growing? If you see the shiny or "silvery" side of the grass, it means that the grass is growing away from you, so it will be fast—fast as quicksilver. If the dull side of the grass is facing you, a harder putt will be necessary, because the grain will slow the ball.

If the shine is on the right side of your projected putt, aim a bit to the left of where you think you should. If the shine is to the left, aim a bit farther to the right.

If you are near water, the grass will tend to grow toward the water, so it will be faster putting toward the water. This is often true even if the water is miles away. For example, at Riviera Country Club in Los Angeles, the course is several miles from the ocean, but the ball always seems to break toward the ocean.

Another factor that can affect the way the grass will play is the amount of dampness from rain, fog, or recent watering. The dampness factor affects your putt by slowing it down and making it break less than you might expect.

The wind tends to flatten the grass and make the ball break in the direction that the wind is blowing. And if the wind has been blowing for some time, it has probably dried out the greens and made them faster, which will make the breaking putt break more than expected.

Reading the Slope

It is equally important to read the slope. On hilly courses the ball will generally break away from the hill. The green may look flat to the naked eye, but the contour of the hill generally masks the true slope of the putting surface.

One of the best methods of correctly reading an unfamiliar green is the plumb-bob method. First, you must establish which of your eyes is your domi-

Reading the slope

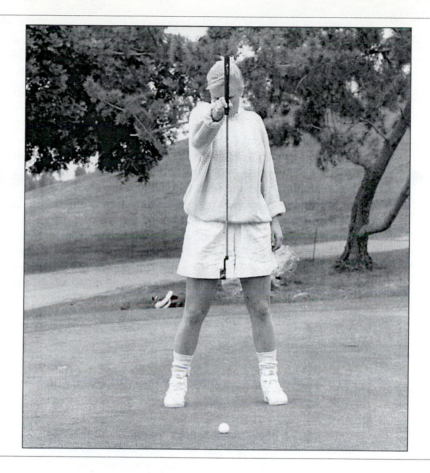

nant eye. You can do this by looking at a narrow object some distance away. Now with your fist clenched and at arm's length, stick up your thumb and block out the object with your thumb. With both eyes open you should not be able to see the object. Now close your right eye, then open it. Next close your left eye, then open it. With one eye the object will be visible, and with the other it will be covered. The eye that cannot see the object is your dominant eye, because it was the eye that controlled your vision when you looked with two eyes.

Next, hold up your putter in line with a perpendicular object—perhaps a fence post or edge of a building. While looking with your dominant eye and with your putter hanging freely between your thumb and index finger, move the putter in your hand until it is parallel with the perpendicular object. Remember where you grip it in order to make it hang vertically every time you want to use this method. You won't always have a vertical post on the course by which to plumb your bob.

Now that the putter is hanging vertically, step behind the ball. Spread your feet and straighten your legs. (This will stop you from compensating for a sloping green by bending one knee.) Line up the bottom of your putter shaft with the center of the ball. If the hole appears on the right side of the upper part of the putter shaft, the putt will break right. If it is on the left side, it will break left.

Generally, if the hole appeared 10 inches to the right of your putter shaft, you should aim your putt 10 inches to the left and let it break right toward the hole.

Combining Your Reads

The next step is to combine your reads. To arrive at the perfect putt for a situation, you have to figure the combined effect of the slope of the green, the lay of the grass grain, the wetness or dryness of the surface, and the distance of the putt.

For example, if you are putting uphill into the wind, but the grain of the grass is growing away from you, as it often does at the ocean, the wind and the uphill putt will be nearly cancelled out by the grain of the grass.

One last thought on breaking putts comes to us from a study done on tournament players by the British Golf Society. It showed that 85 percent of breaking putts were missed below the hole. This means the professionals were reading less break into the greens than was actually there. When you miss, are you above or below the hole most of the time?

The Alignment Mode

Your alignment mode now must be figured. Here is where you combine your reads and predict the path of the ball. Visualize the putt that you want to make, considering the slope, the grain, the wind, and the dampness factors. If the green is flat, see it go straight to the hole. If the green is undulating, see it curve along the break that you have decided it must make.

After you have decided just how much break you will allow on the putt, pick your target. If the cup is within 10 feet, you might aim at the cup or a few inches away to allow for the expected break. On a long putt, of 30 or more feet, you must putt at a target rather than the hole. Squat down behind the ball and see the line of the break you expect from the ball. Now pick out a target on that break line about 6 to 10 feet away. Perhaps there is a lighter or darker spot on the grass along that break line. Use that spot for your target.

The Power Mode

Your next decision is the power mode you will use. Decide how far back you will bring your putter to give you enough power to get the ball about 18 inches past the cup. Never putt short and waste a chance of dropping the putt. You should remember that on very long putts, distance is more important than exact accuracy. If your distance will bring you within 10 feet of the cup, you have a chance to "get down in two." But if you are way over or way under, you will still have a long second putt.

Take the proper grip and stance behind the ball. Physically practice your backswing and putting stroke. Your power mode is now settled.

Checklist for Reading the Green

1. Line up your putt while your partners are lining up theirs. Look at the slope of the green and the grain of the grass.

2. Look at the putt from behind the hole. Pace off the distance from the hole to the ball to give you an idea of how hard to stroke.

3. Look at the putt from behind the ball, looking toward the hole. If the grain looks shiny or silvery, the grass is growing away from you, so the putt will be faster than normal. If the grain of the grass looks dull, it is growing toward you and will slow down your putt. Grass generally grows toward the west.

4. Read the slope of the green from ahead, behind, and below the path of the putt. Remember that the green generally slopes away from a mountain or hill—even if it looks flat.

5. Watch your partners' putts. Is the green fast or slow? Does it have a break that you did not expect? Pay particular attention to any putt that is on the same line as yours.

6. If you are unsure of the break on a short putt, hit the ball reasonably hard to the center of the hole. This will reduce the break that is increased with a slower putt.

Making the Putt

To make the putt, line up your putter blade perpendicular to the line of putt that you want—the line between your ball and your target. Look at a small spot on the back of the ball. Take your putter back as far as you have physically practiced. Then move it through the ball smoothly. And watch the ball settle into the cup.

If you are within 2 feet of the cup, you can putt out without waiting your turn. Always do this. The odds are with you if you confidently putt out rather than waiting and trying to read the break in this mini-putt. Chances are you will just confuse yourself.

Putting Etiquette

Putting etiquette requires that you not bother your partners with noise or movement and that you keep the greens in top condition. Place your clubs on the far side of the green near the next tee. Never lay your clubs on the green, and never roll a cart across the green. The putting surface is so fragile that the weight of the clubs or cart can cause depressions in the grass that may hinder a following player.

Repairing a divot on the green

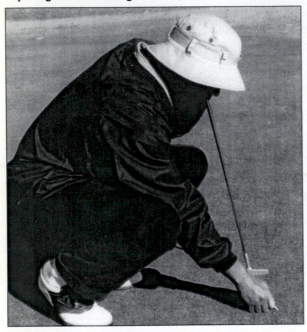

Slide a tee under the depression

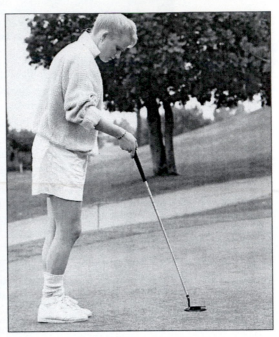

Gently tamp it down with your putter

Etiquette on the putting surface

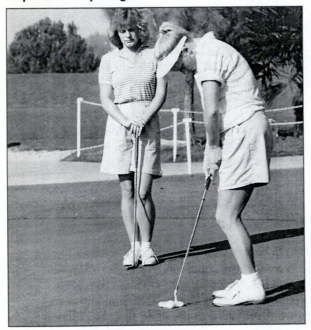

Do not stand directly behind the putting player

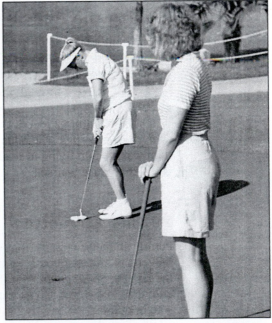

Do not stand in line with the putt in front of the player

Etiquette also requires that you repair the greens when necessary. When a ball has hit the green and left a depression (divot) slide your forked green-repair tool or a long tee under the depression and lift the turf gently until it is even with the surrounding grass. Then gently tamp it down with your putter blade to make certain that it is not higher than the surrounding area.

Remember that the player farthest from the hole putts first. Also, line up your putt when your partners are lining up theirs, then stand away from the person who is putting—preferably facing him or her. Standing in line with the putt, either near the hole or behind the putting player, may cause a distraction.

 ## Checklist for Etiquette on the Greens

1. Mark your ball on the green so that it will not be in the line of sight of another player who is putting.
2. If your ball is closest to the hole, tend the pin or pull it out on request and lay it down on the putting surface.
3. If you lay the pin down on the green, make sure that it is not in the line of sight of another player who is putting.
4. Do not step in the line of another player's putt between the ball and the hole.
5. Do not stand behind a player who is putting. Stay away from his or her line of sight. (The best place to stand is face to face with the player who is putting.)
6. Line your putt up while the other players in your foursome are lining up theirs, and be ready to putt when it is your turn.
7. Do not move around while another player is putting.
8. Do not talk while another player is putting.
9. Move your ball marker if it is in the line of another player's putt.
10. Take your ball out of the hole after you have completed your putt.
11. Make certain that your shadow does not fall across the ball, the hole, or the line of another player's putt.
12. Do not leave the green until all of the members of your foursome have putted out.
13. Repair all ball marks on the green.
14. When you are tending the pin, make certain that your shadow does not fall across the hole or across the line of the putt.

✓   *Checklist for Repairing a Ball Mark*

1. Bring the soil around the ball mark upward into the center of the mark by sticking a repair tool or a tee under the mark and pushing upward gently.
2. Tap the raised area back down with your putter so that it is even with the surrounding turf.
3. Repair only the ball marks that are on your putting line.
4. Repair spike marks anywhere on the green.
5. Do not hold up play by remaining on the green to repair any marks after your foursome has putted.
6. Repair marks only while your partners are lining up their putts, not while they are putting.

Summary

1. Putting is perhaps the most important part of the game. A 1-inch putt into the hole counts one stroke just as does a 400-yard drive off the tee does.
2. You should read the greens as thoroughly as possible, figuring the line of your putt and the amount of power needed. This will give you confidence.
3. Physically practice the power phase of your stroke before you address the ball. Take a solid stance, with your eyes over the ball. Stroke the ball while accelerating the clubhead through it.
4. Proper etiquette is essential on the green.

9

Plotting Your Strategy on the Course

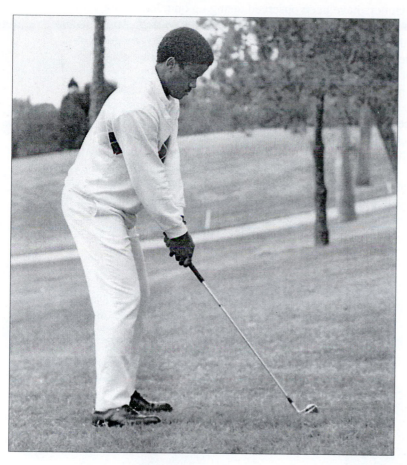

Outline

Club Selection

Proper club selection is essential to a good game of golf. Most beginners consistently choose a shorter (higher-numbered) club than they should and therefore rarely hit the ball as long as they need to. So if you are a beginner, remember to choose "enough club" to get the job done. Most greens have trouble in the front not the back, so it's generally better to hit on or over the green than to come up short in a trap.

Beware of the temptation to use a "favorite" club instead of the proper club for the shot. Beginners have been observed teeing up on a long par 4 with a favorite club—a 5-iron, for example. A par is impossible with that type of club selection. Play the game the way it is meant to be played. On any given day, you may be able to drive better than you expect to, hit a second good shot, and be on the green in 2.

Although there are times when it is better to play it safe by choosing a lesser club in order to win a hole or a match, when you are playing just for fun it is a good idea to see what you can do by playing a longer club. That way you will have a much better idea of what to expect from each of your clubs.

The driver, the wedge, and the putter are the most important clubs in your bag. They don't have to go with the balanced set of clubs you use for the rest of your game. Anytime you find a driver that works well for you, buy it. Try several drivers until you find one you can hit well. The driver is probably the most important club in the bag. While putting is the most important skill, it doesn't do you much good to 1-putt if you have hit the ball out of bounds or in the water a couple of times.

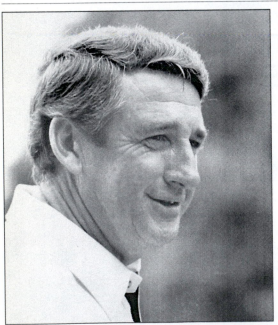

J. C. Says

"When I first started on the tour, I got to play with Sam, Bob Goalby, Miller Barber. I would go over to them and ask them what clubs they were playing and why. What the percentages were, etc.

Even today on the tour I will walk over to another player and look in his bag to see what clubs he's hitting with. The reason for their use may indicate something he's figured out about the course. If you put other player's reasoning into your mental golf bag, it might save you a shot or win you a tournament sometime."

These two holes, though similar, require different strategies

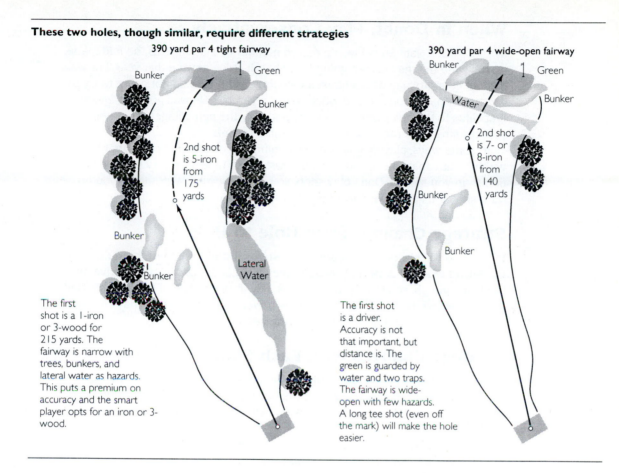

390 yard par 4 tight fairway

Bunker

Green

Bunker

2nd shot is 5-iron from 175 yards

Bunker

Bunker

Lateral Water

The first shot is a 1-iron or 3-wood for 215 yards. The fairway is narrow with trees, bunkers, and lateral water as hazards. This puts a premium on accuracy and the smart player opts for an iron or 3-wood.

390 yard par 4 wide-open fairway

Bunker

Green

Water

Bunker

2nd shot is 7- or 8-iron from 140 yards

Bunker

Bunker

The first shot is a driver. Accuracy is not that important, but distance is. The green is guarded by water and two traps. The fairway is wide-open with few hazards. A long tee shot (even off the mark) will make the hole easier.

Before choosing your club, you must determine your first-shot strategy. Will you go for the perfect shot or the high-percentage shot? Rather than playing for the perfect shot, as so many amateurs do, ask yourself a few questions. Can I play this low-percentage shot by hitting a driver down a tight fairway and try for a birdie? Or do I hit an iron off the tee and then hit a longer shot to the green? This way I may get a par. You won't get as many birdies playing it safe, but your average scores will be lower.

Certain holes may shake your confidence. In that event, use a 1-iron or 2-iron and settle for keeping the ball in play. Your feelings may even vary from day to day. On a cold or windy day or when you feel tight, you might elect to play a lesser club than on a calm day or on a day when you feel like you can't do anything wrong.

Just because a hole is a par-4 or a par-5 doesn't mean you have to use a driver; and if you choose to drive, you don't necessarily have to give it everything you've got.

When in Doubt, Play Conservatively

In 1950, when Sam Snead won a record number of tournaments, he had made up his mind that he was not going to try to out-drive anyone that year, but was instead going to play within himself the whole year. He was not going to try to get on any par-5 holes in two when it was a gamble. He was going to *lay up* (get close to the hole) when necessary and play the percentages. That was the year his stroke average was 69.23. It is still a record.

In some ways, playing golf is like gambling. If you play the odds (that is, within your capabilities), you will win most of the time. Don't try to drive farther than you should. Don't play shots you can't execute. Why should you go for a shot you can make only one out of ten times?

Strategy Changes from Hole to Hole

In winning the playoff against Seve Ballesteros in the 1987 Westchester Classic, J.C. Snead won the draw and chose to tee off second. Seve hit a bad drive into the heavy rough, so J.C. played a 4-iron safely in the middle of the fairway. Had J.C. drawn first, he would have hit a long driver. So your strategy may change very abruptly depending on the circumstances.

Strategy Changes with Each Shot

There is a time to gamble and a time to play it safe. For example, in the tall grass you cannot control the spin of the ball well, so take one more club than necessary for that distance, then choke down on it. This way you are not as likely to hit flyers.

There are players on the tour with great swings who hit all their practice shots like champs, but don't know how to play the shots on the course. They don't know which club to use or where to try to place the ball. Consequently, their great swings are of little benefit to them against players who understand strategy.

On any shot to the green, even with a wedge, check the pin placement. If the pin is to the right of the green, aim to the left. At least you can plan on being on the green. If you aim slightly to the "fat" side of the pin, you can avoid the possible trouble near the edge of the green.

One of the first things to learn in golf strategy is acceptance of the need to take an extra stroke to compensate for a bad shot. If you are in the woods, just chip back out on the fairway and play your next shot. There is no sense in trying to hit a 2-iron through a keyhole to get closer to the green. You would be surprised at how many times you can save par if you play conservatively. Since the odds are against you in the woods, you are wiser to take your sure shot out than to try to save a stroke by aiming toward the hole and probably hitting two trees, a squirrel, and ending up out of bounds. Discretion is the better part of valor.

Strategy changes with every shot. You can't, for example, plan from the tee to play a shot 5 yards inside the right-hand bunker, then hit a 4-iron to within 10 feet of the pin on the downhill side, then 2-putt. What if you hit into the bunker or land in the rough? Then your strategy must change. Every shot calls into play new strategy. You play one shot at a time, not one hole at a time.

Many times when you warm up on the practice tee, you find that you are hitting the ball a certain way—right or left, long or short. Take that lesson with you to the first tee. Don't fight what you are tending to do that day. If you are playing well, but your shots are going generally left to right, plan that into your strategy. Start from the right side of the tee and aim left. You might hit too far right, but at least you have an idea of about where the ball is likely to go.

Your strategic decisions must take into account what you are doing well and what you are doing poorly on a given day. If you try to correct what is natural for you at that time, you may create more problems. Work with what you have. After the round, you might try to straighten out the problem on the practice tee. But during the round, play the percentages.

When you get on the tee, look at the hole to determine the best way to play it depending on where the trouble is. Then, if you don't make your shot exactly the way you planned, change your strategy. You can't plan every shot in advance.

There is no set way to play any hole. Sometimes you will hit a great drive, hit your second shot on the green, and 1-putt, and you will say, "That was easy. That's the way that hole ought to have been played." On other days, however, that same hole will require a different strategy. On the days when everything is going your way and you are "on your game," your strategy will be different than on the days when you are "off your game."

✔ *Checklist for Golf Strategy*

1. Use the high-percentage shot off of the tee rather than trying to hit the ball for distance only.
2. Use an iron to tee off on a tight fairway.
3. Always be aware of wind and weather conditions, and play your shot accordingly.
4. Always use "enough club" to make the shot required. Avoid the temptation to hit your "perfect" shot with a lesser club.
5. Avoid the temptation to try to make a "career shot" when you are in trouble. Play it safe and get the ball out of trouble first!
6. When in doubt, play conservatively. The odds are with you.
7. Know the rules! Know *when* and *where* you can drop the ball for relief. Know the local rules also.
8. Always play a provisional ball if you think your first ball is lost or out of bounds.
9. Always read the grain as well as the break on the putting green, especially at a seaside course.
10. Always watch how your playing partner's ball breaks on the putting green, especially when the putt is on the same line as yours.

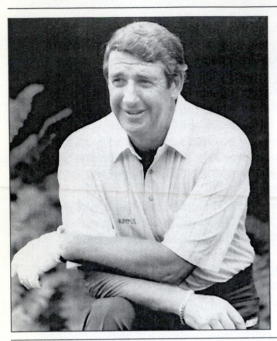

J.C. Says:

"Some of the amateurs we play with are so conscious of their grip, stance, and swing that they forget to look to see where they are going. They must stand up and hit it. Another thing amateurs often do is hit right into a tree in the center of the fairway. It's amazing to see what people will do to waste strokes."

Summary

1. Every day that you play you should have a general strategy for the overall approach to your game.

2. Do you want to gamble, trying for the perfect shot on every swing? Then attempt your "hero" shots. Or do you want to win the match? Then play the game close to the vest, because the odds are with the tortoise, not the hare.

3. Choose the club that will send the ball as far as you want it. Many beginners hit too short.

4. Be prepared to change your strategy from hole to hole and from shot to shot.

10 *A Strategy for Each Hole*

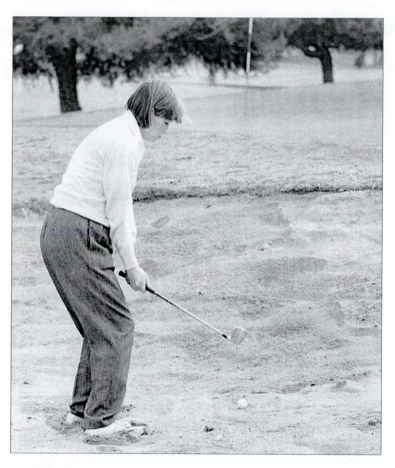

Outline

E ach hole requires a different strategy, since each presents a different set of challenges—in the form of distance, shape of fairway, and trees and other hazards.

3-Par Holes

Three par holes look easy because they are short, but they are often designed to be extra difficult. They may be uphill or downhill, over a water hazard, have small greens, or be heavily trapped. Consequently, accuracy, not power, is your major concern with a 3-par hole.

If it only a short to mid-iron shot seems necessary, the hole is a possible *birdie* hole. But always play the percentages. Aim the ball at the center of the green, unless you are a *fader*, in which case you should stand on the right side of the tee and aim down the left side of the green. You'll be surprised at how many greens you can hit by this approach.

Selecting the Right Club off the Tee

First read the sign that tells you the distance from the tee to the hole. What iron or wood will you need for that distance? Then consider any obstacles on the hole and adjust your decision accordingly. Let's assume that the hole is 170 yards and that you would normally play a 4-iron for that distance. If there is water or a sand trap in front of the green but nothing behind the green, you might opt for 3-iron instead, and play it easy. The same might be true if the pin is placed deep on the green. What if the hole is uphill? Perhaps you will want a 3-iron or 2-iron, since you always need "more club" when shooting uphill. Conversely, if the hole is downhill, you would use "less club," perhaps a 5-iron or a 6-iron.

Play your strengths. Hit the shot you are confident about. Don't be afraid to "lay the ball up" short of the green, avoiding the traps, then chip up close to the pin. Make your strategic decisions conservative, and you will have much more confidence.

Once you have decided where you want to hit the ball and have selected your club, have faith in your decision. You probably made the best choice. Be confident. Regard that club as your friend. You chose it. Trust it to do its job well.

Teeing Up

If your ball tends to *fade* (go to the right rather than straight), you should always favor the right side of the tee, then hit left. This way, when the ball fades, it will come back to where you want it. Conversely, if you hit a draw (the ball curves left), line up on the left of the tee and hit right. With this strategy, the ball should be working toward the hole after it lands on the green.

Tee box positioning based on your shot tendencies

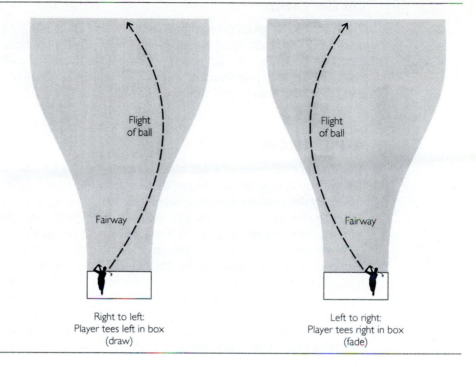

Right to left:
Player tees left in box
(draw)

Left to right:
Player tees right in box
(fade)

Use a tee for a 3-par hole. There is no reason to hit off the grass just because you are using an iron. You will have a much better chance of making a good shot by using a tee. And you will be amazed at what that tee will do for your confidence. Tee the ball up just above grass level, but no higher. If you tee too high, you may pop it up and waste your shot.

Use a good ball. If you play an old ball just in case it goes into that water hazard, you are conceding defeat before you begin.

Approach Shot

Let's assume that you didn't land the ball on the green with your tee shot. You will undoubtedly use a wedge for your second shot. Gauge the distance and the slope of the green. Remember, you want to land your ball on the green. If the pin is set near the fringe, don't try to get too close to the pin and risk having your ball roll off the green.

Visualize how far back you will take your club. Visualize your whole shot. Take your practice swing, incorporating everything you just visualized. Step up to the ball, aim, and make your shot.

On the Green

If you are on the green on your first shot, you are "on in one." All you have to do is 2-putt for a par. Read the green from both sides of the hole. Pace off your putt. Plan on having enough power in your stroke to roll the ball 2 feet past the hole. Line up your putt. Practice your stroke while you visualize sinking the putt. Take your stance, and sink your putt.

4-Par Holes

The special challenges of 4-par holes generally lie in a narrow fairway, which can get you in trouble on your tee shot, or a change in direction—a dogleg. Generally the person who hits straight does best on a 4-par hole. It is always better to play the percentages, so if the hole is 390 yards and you hit 220 yards with a 1-iron, you should plan on using a 5-iron or 6-iron shot to the green.

When teeing up, look at the design of the hole, then look at the best way to play your shot. Go with the grain. The newer courses often don't give you a true picture of the design of the hole. Sometimes you can't even see the fairway. For these courses, you may find it best to pick out something in the distance, such as a building or a tree, and try to hit at that target rather than looking at the ground and the way it slopes. Then once you get near the green, you can get a better feel of the area and will know better how to hit your approach shot.

If your fairway is very narrow, conservative strategy dictates that you use a club that you can control when teeing off. The 3-wood might be a good choice. If you are playing a dogleg, you have the option of (1) trying to go for distance and straighten out the curve or (2) playing it safe to avoid trouble. On a dogleg to the left, you might tee up on the left of the tee and hit into the center of the fairway, or you could tee up on the right and try to straighten out the dogleg.

On a long 4-par, the best you can hope for is to be on the green in two. The question is whether you want to play your drive safe by making your approach with a longer iron, or straighten out the fairway (hit closer to the angle of the dogleg) and hope you will have a shorter iron shot to the green. So while you would like to drive the ball long, if there is a blind side or a tree hanging out, you will need the control of a lesser club.

Above all else, play it safe enough to avoid the fairway bunkers. Don't try to get all the distance possible by hitting too hard. Hit the ball straight and stay out of trouble.

REMEMBER THAT THE ODDS ARE WITH YOU WHEN YOUR STRATEGY IS TO PLAY IT SAFE AND YOUR TECHNIQUE IS TO SWING EASY!

What if your tee shot goes into the trees? If no high-percentage shot through the trees is possible, use your wedge to pitch the ball out on the fairway. It's

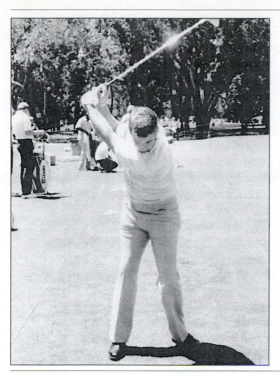

J. C. Says

"On real tight par-4s under 395 yards, a low-handicapper might hit a 1-iron or a 2-iron off the tee. Most people can hit an iron straighter than a wood. And if you hit the ball straight, you will be better off. Distance is not always the most important thing. If you can hit long and straight consistently, you will out-hit any of us on the tour."

surprising how often those trees want to get into your game and hit your ball. So as long as they didn't pay your greens fees, don't let the forest into your foursome.

In order to reach the green, it is often a good idea, on your second shot, to take one more club than you think you need, a 4-iron rather than a 5-iron. Then swing easy. You will be amazed at how accurate you can be if you don't try to force it. Actually, if your tee shot is effective, the rest of the hole is like playing a 3-par.

5-Par Holes

As we said earlier, you should always plot your strategy for a hole before you tee off. So the first thing you must do on a 5-par is to check the drawing on the scorecard. Where is the trouble? Are there hazards on the fairway? Do you have a chance to be on in two, or should you plan on laying up your second shot short of the green and the traps that guard it? How do you want to hit your tee shot?

Once you have formed a mental picture of the hole and how you will play it, select your tee spot. Always tee up close to trouble and hit away from it. So if the water or bunkers are on the left, tee up left, and hit toward the right of the fairway.

The 5-par requires that you hit for both distance and placement on your first two shots. But if there is a choice between distance or accuracy, always go with accuracy.

In selecting your tee spot, look for a level area between the tee markers or back as far as two club lengths; you have a choice of any place within an area of about 20 to 30 square yards. Tee the ball up so that at least half of the ball is above the top of the driver when the clubhead is resting on the ground. If you are playing into the wind, however, and you want to hit the ball low, you should tee the ball down a little bit. If you want to hit it high, tee it higher.

Once you have teed up, pick your target area. Don't think about avoiding an area, such as a water hazard; but rather, concentrate on hitting an area that you have chosen. Think positively on the golf course.

When you have selected your target area, stand behind your tee and mentally rehearse your shot. Then take three deep breaths if you need to relax. Take your practice swing. Then take your stance and address the ball, concentrate on a spot on the back side of the ball, and make your shot.

If you can control the ball well, work the ball away from trouble. Thus, if you have a lake on the left and a dogleg on the right, tee up on the right side and aim down the left side to make the ball turn away from the water. The same holds true for fairway bunkers. Work the ball away from them. They are difficult for most people, so we suggest that you stay out of them.

If the hole is a par-5 with a dogleg right and bunkers on the right, keep the ball to the left. Play into the fat part of the dogleg. This is even more important on a 5-par than on a 4-par hole. It is often a good idea to hit short of the bunker, then lay up from there with a club you can control, since on par-5 holes you probably can't reach the green on your second shot.

There is no sense in hitting a 3-wood for a second shot, because it's probably the hardest club to control. Instead, take a long iron that you can control (a 3-, 4-, or 5-iron), and try to get close to the green. The 3-wood might work well if there is no trouble ahead—no water, bunkers, or out-of-bounds. However, there is no point in using a 3-wood to try to clear the water with a 230-yard shot. Amateurs sometimes try to make their career shot in such a situation, but they would be far wiser to use a club that they know they can hit 150 yards or better with, and then hit down the fairway short of the trouble. This will leave an 8-iron or 9-iron shot to the green.

Strategy for a 5-par hole might start with answering the question of where you would like to make your third shot. How can you get near that point while avoiding the hazards of the fairway and the out-of-bounds?

A sample 5-par hole is seen on the next page. The diagram illustrates how three players with varying abilities might decide to play this tough 5-par. Each player develops a strategy based on his or her own strengths and weaknesses. Each player faces the same dilemmas. How close does one play to the hazards on the left on the tee shot? Is it wise to attempt a second shot to the green, or is it better to lay up for an easy third shot?

Here you would want to tee up on the left to avoid the fairway bunkers on the left. Aim toward the right side of the fairway. Place the ball with confidence. For your second shot, you can play a wood or an iron, because you want to lay up short of the traps that guard the green.

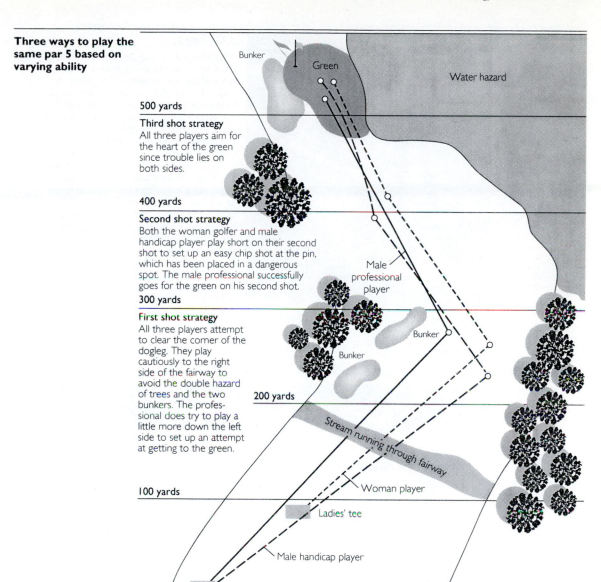

Three ways to play the same par 5 based on varying ability

Bunker

Green

Water hazard

500 yards

Third shot strategy
All three players aim for the heart of the green since trouble lies on both sides.

400 yards

Second shot strategy
Both the woman golfer and male handicap player play short on their second shot to set up an easy chip shot at the pin, which has been placed in a dangerous spot. The male professional successfully goes for the green on his second shot.

300 yards

First shot strategy
All three players attempt to clear the corner of the dogleg. They play cautiously to the right side of the fairway to avoid the double hazard of trees and the two bunkers. The professional does try to play a little more down the left side to set up an attempt at getting to the green.

Male professional player

Bunker

Bunker

200 yards

Stream running through fairway

100 yards

Woman player

Ladies' tee

Male handicap player

Men's tee

Playing Around the Greens on 4-Pars and 5-Pars

Strategy for playing long 4-pars or short 5-pars will depend on pin placement. If the pin is in the back, and you have no bunkers to go over, and you are about 10 yards off the green, you can use a less lofted club. Chip-and-run with a 7-iron or 8-iron. But if the pin is set close, and you don't have much green to work with, you should pitch with your sand wedge or pitching wedge.

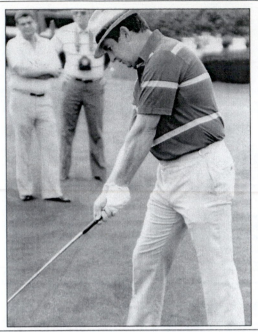

J.C. Says:

"The 18th hole at Augusta is a fairly long uphill hole. You can try to drive it or lay up. A lot of the tour players will try to lay up with a 3-wood. You can tee up right and play to the left and fade away from the traps. If you draw, tee up left and hit right. It is not a good hole to draw on. It is better to hit straight. Just make sure that you take the traps out of play.

After your tee shot you can be left with a 165- or 170-yard shot up the hill. You might use a 7-iron to a front pin placement or a 5-iron to a back pin placement. If you can't get the ball to the green on the fly, the best strategy is to play it up the right side. Run it up into the mouth of the green and play for the birdie or the easy par. If you are a long ways from the pin, it is a very difficult hole to 2-putt. It has an undulating green and is usually slick. Any time you can put the ball in the middle of this green, you are doing a pretty good job."

✓ Checklist for Teeing Up the Ball

1. If using a driver, tee the ball so that half of the ball is above the top of the club-head of the driver.
2. If using a fairway wood on the tee, tee the ball lower than you would for a driver.
3. If using an iron on the tee, the ball should set just above the turf.
4. Look for a level area on the tee so that your lie and your stance will be level.

Summary

1. Each type of hole has its own set of challenges, according to the distance factor, the shape of the fairway, and the trees and other hazards. A positive mental attitude can minimize the dangers of these pitfalls.

2. In developing our strategies, we become the quarterback for our golf game. It is the constant mental challenge that makes it a great sport. Three keys to success are as follows:

   - Play conservatively.
   - Choose the club that will do the job.
   - Think positively. Concentrate on where you want the shot to land, not on where you don't want to hit it, such as in a pond or bunker.

11   *The Rules of Golf*

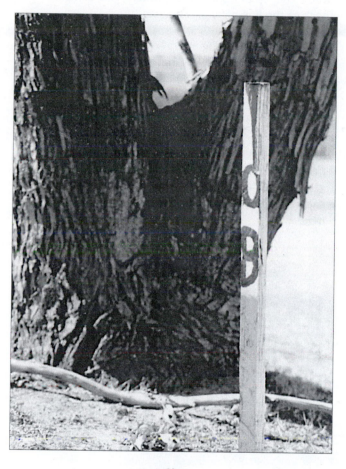

Outline

On the Tee

The ball must be teed up between the tee markers. There may be two or three sets of tee markers. The tee markers closest to the hole are called the *front* tees and are usually played by players who do not hit a long ball. Many women, youths, and senior citizens will play from the front tees. The next tees back are the *regular* tees. If there is a third tee area farther from the pin, it is called the *championship* or *back* tee.

Although you are not allowed to tee up in front of the markers, you can go as far back as two club lengths from the line between the tees.

If the ball falls off the tee before you have started forward with your swing, you may replace it without a penalty. If you miss the ball completely, it is called a *whiff*, and you must count it as a stroke. If you hit the ball any distance, even 1 inch, your stroke counts and you must play the ball where it lies.

Scoring

Each hit ball, whiff, and penalty is included in the score as a stroke. In *match play* the strokes are counted for each hole, and the winner of that hole is determined. The winner of the competition is the person who has won the most holes. In *stroke play* the total number of strokes for the round determines the winner. Most rounds are 18 holes.

You can tee off anywhere within the rectangle formed by two clubs and the tee markers

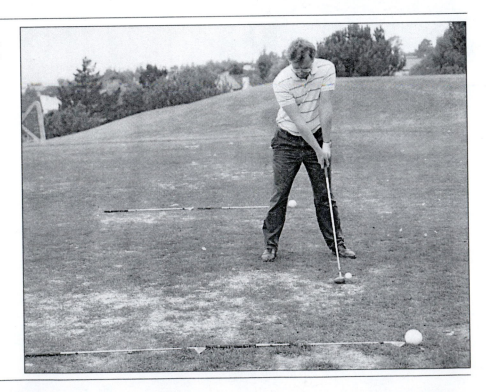

**The order of play
after teeing off**   Player A is away, then C and then B

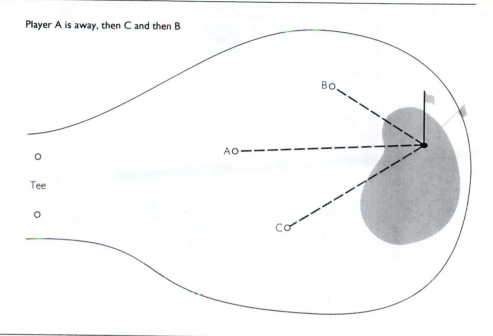

Order of Play

After the tee shot, the person farthest from the green always hits first. This is called "being away," meaning that person is the farthest away from the hole.

Playing the Ball

The object of golf is to "play the ball as it lies." The game pits you against the course. Though there are provisions for you to play a different lie under some circumstances, you receive penalty strokes for taking advantage of such provisions.

Some courses allow you to move the ball up to 6 inches in playing *winter rules*. These so-called "rules" are not sanctioned by the official rules of golf, so do not get into the habit of playing by them.

There are times when you must *drop the ball* before you can hit it. Certain man-made hazards are noted in the official rules as justification for doing this. You pick up the ball, stand up straight, holding the ball at arm's length at your side, then drop it. If the ball rolls more than two club lengths, closer to the cup, out of bounds, into a hazard, or touches a player or a player's equipment, it must be dropped again.

If you lose your ball and cannot find it within five minutes, allow the players following to *play through*. If you still cannot find your ball, take a one-stroke

Dropping the ball

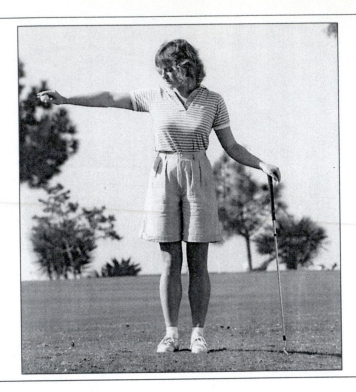

penalty and go back to the place from where you hit your last shot and hit another ball. If it was your tee shot that was lost, you may tee the ball again. If the original ball is found later, you must continue to play the second ball and count your penalty stroke.

If you hit out of bounds, count that shot, add another for a penalty, then hit a second ball from where you hit the shot that went out of bounds. You will have used three strokes instead of just one.

A *provisional ball* can be hit if you think that your ball may be lost or out of bounds. You must tell your playing partners that you are hitting a provisional ball. If you find that your original ball was out of bounds, give yourself a penalty stroke. (You would now be "lying three." Count your original stroke that went out of bounds, your penalty stroke, and your provisional ball stroke.) If you find that your original ball was in bounds, just pick up your provisional ball and go on playing, not counting the stroke that you hit for the provisional ball. You are not allowed to hit a provisional ball if your first shot went into a water hazard.

If you hit the wrong ball, except in a hazard, you lose the hole in match play, or two strokes in stroke play. (There is no penalty if you hit the wrong ball in a hazard.)

> ✓ *Checklist for Finding a Lost Ball*
>
> 1. On the tee, each player should follow each tee shot and note where a shot may have gone into the rough by noting a tree or other marker.
> 2. Listen for the sound of a ball hitting a tree or water.
> 3. When you have determined where a lost ball probably lies, start there and then expand your search in an orderly manner.
> 4. Allow a following group to play through if you are delaying them by looking for a ball.
> 5. Never search for more than five minutes.
> 6. If you cannot find the ball, go back to the spot where you hit the lost ball and hit another shot, and assess yourself a penalty stroke.
> 7. Know the brand and number of the ball you hit so that you can identify it if someone finds a ball.

Unplayable Lies

If you decide that your ball is unplayable (because it is next to a tree, or in the water, for example), you may take a one-stroke penalty and replay the shot from where you originally hit it. (This is a total of three strokes, counting your original shot, the penalty, and your second shot.) Or you can take a two-stroke penalty and drop the ball anywhere along the line from where you originally hit it to where it lies unplayable. (In which case, you will be lying three on that shot.) Keep the pin in line with the ball.

Sometimes man-made problems (like benches, hoses, or ground under repair) or acts of God (like a rain that left water where it was not supposed to be—called *casual water*) make your shot difficult. Here you can improve your lie by either moving the problems (such as a hose) or dropping the ball from a spot within one club length of the nearest *point of relief* (the closest area from which it might be played). The ball must not roll more than two club lengths, or it must be dropped again.

Obstructions are anything that might interfere with your swing or your shot but are not part of the course design. If your ball lands next to a machine, rest-room, snack stand, a sprinkler head, an immovable bench, or other such obstruction, you can move the ball to the nearest point of relief, as long as it is not nearer the hole, and drop it within one club length of that point.

Suppose you encounter an obstruction such as a young tree that is being supported by wires held by stakes. If your ball falls within that area, you can bring it out to the closest area from which it might be played (the point of relief), then drop it one club length farther from that point.

Out-of-bounds are clearly marked with white stakes

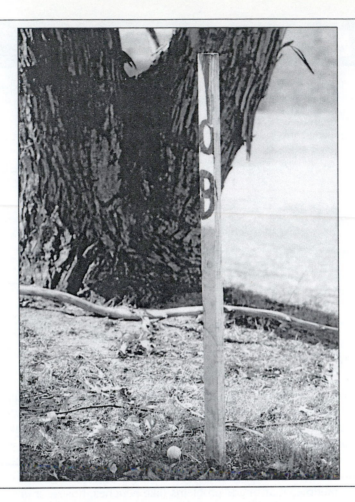

Not everything that obstructs your swing is an obstruction. An unstaked tree, low branches, long grass, rocks, or divot holes are considered part of the course, so if your ball lands near them, you have to play it as it lies.

Ground under repair may be indicated by a sign when the ground is being newly seeded or plowed. If your ball lands in such an area, you can pick it up and drop it within one club length of the nearest point of relief that is not nearer the hole. If there is no sign for the ground under repair, you can move the ball as long as your opponents agree. If you are playing in a tournament, the tournament committee must approve your moving the ball.

As explained before, casual water is any water that was not designed into the course. A puddle left from a rain or the lawn sprinklers would be an example. If you find yourself in casual water, you can move the ball to the nearest point of relief, then drop it one club length from that point (no nearer to the hole). If you encounter casual water in a trap, you can either move the ball

**An unplayable lie is a
one-stroke penalty**

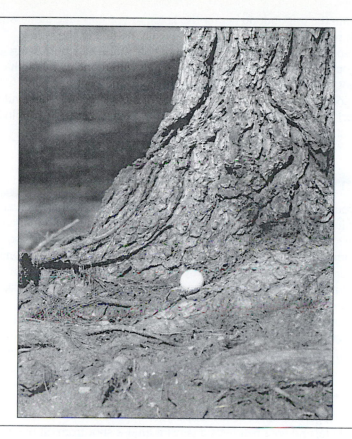

 Checklist for Taking Relief

1. Know the rule for dropping the ball for relief without penalty.
2. Be alert to taking relief from cart paths, casual water, or ground under repair. If any of them interfere with your stance, your swing, or the lie of the ball, you can take relief.
3. When taking relief, drop your ball one club length from the problem that allows you relief.
4. You may clean your ball before dropping it.
5. If you have difficulty in determining the point from which you will mark the one club length for relief, mark the spot with a tee before measuring.
6. Check your scorecard to determine whether there are local rules that allow relief in special situations, such as when you are in a drainage ditch or next to a fence.

within the trap (but no nearer the hole), or you can take a one-stroke penalty and remove the ball from the trap (again, no nearer the hole).

Sometimes your ball will land in a hole made by a burrowing animal such as a gopher or mole. If so, just drop the ball within one club length of the nearest point of relief that is not closer to the hole, and continue play.

Local rules are printed on the back of the scorecard. These rules will explain specific penalties or situations particular to that course. If you find yourself in a questionable situation, consult the local rules first.

On the Green

If you want to remove your ball from where it lies so that you can clean it or get it out of the way of another player's putting line, put a marker, such as a dime, directly behind the ball and then pick up the ball. If it is still in the line of another player's putt, move the marker one putter head away and remark it. When it is your turn to putt, move it back to its original position.

If another player's ball lies near your line of putt, you may ask your opponent to mark the spot and pick up the ball. It is your decision.

You can have the pin in or out of the hole or *tended*, meaning that another player holds the pin until you have completed your stroke. In stroke play, if you hit the tended pin or the player holding it, you take a two-stroke penalty. You also take a two-stroke penalty if you putt into a pin lying on the ground. (There is no penalty for hitting the pin from a shot made from off the green.)

In match play, if you hit the pin that your opponent laid down, or if you hit your opponent or his or her clubs, your opponent wins the hole. If the pin is in the hole, and your ball rests against it after a shot from off the green, pull the pin. If the ball drops, you made it. If it rolls away from the cup, you must putt it.

If casual water on the green prevents you from making your putt, you can move the ball to the nearest point of relief, not nearer the hole.

You cannot smooth the ground in the line of your putt, but you can remove loose impediments such as leaves or twigs from the green. If your ball moves while you are moving these things, you lose a stroke.

If you have *holed out*, and your opponent is near the edge of the cup, you can concede the putt in match play. But in stroke play, every shot must be made, and you cannot concede a putt.

If you have hit the ball onto a wrong green, you are not allowed to hit your ball from there. Divots on greens are frowned upon. Just drop your ball off the green at the nearest point of relief that is not nearer the hole, and hit your next shot.

Sometimes a putt stops so close to the hole that you know that your opponent will hole out on the next putt. In match play, or when playing just for recreation, you might say "that's a gimme" or "pick it up" (conceding the putt). As mentioned, this is not legal in stroke play. If your opponent has conceded you a putt in match play, you must nevertheless count one stroke, just as if you had putted it in. Conceding the putt just saves a little time.

Mark your ball on the green with a coin

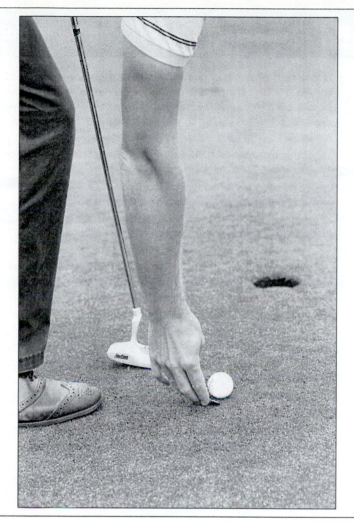

Summary of Penalties

Stroke and Distance Penalties

Lost balls must be replayed from where the original shot was played. You count a stroke for the first shot and a penalty stroke. So your second shot will be counted as if it were your third.

Out-of-bounds balls cannot be played from the out-of-bounds area. Hit another ball from where you hit the one that went out of bounds. Count the first shot and add a penalty stroke. So your second hit will be counted as a third stroke.

Missing the ball or a *whiff* counts as one stroke.

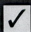 **Checklist on Important Rules of Golf**

1. If you hit the ball out of bounds, you must play another ball from where you hit the first one. The penalty is both for the stroke and the distance. It is one stroke because you hit the ball out of bounds, and another stroke for the distance that you already hit. So you are hitting your third shot after hitting out of bounds, taking the penalty, then hitting again.

2. Your tee shot must be teed up behind the markers and no more than two club lengths behind the markers.

3. If you miss the ball and it falls off the tee, it counts as a stroke. But if you did not cause it to fall off the tee, there is no penalty.

4. If you cause the ball to move when you are lining up a fairway shot or removing impediments around it, you must count it as a stroke.

5. If you are in a hazard, such as a sand trap or water, you cannot move impediments (such as rocks, leaves, and branches) from around the ball.

6. Although you cannot move impediments from around your ball in a hazard, you can remove just enough to identify the ball as yours.

7. The player whose ball is farthest away from the hole hits the next shot.

8. All players should identify their golf balls by brand and number before teeing off on the first hole.

9. Always make certain that the ball you are hitting is yours.

10. Declare a ball lost after searching for five minutes.

11. If a ball is declared lost, the player who lost it must go back to where the last shot was hit and hit another ball. Count one stroke for the shot that was lost and one for having lost it. So the shot being replayed is the third shot.

12. If a player finds the lost ball after having hit a second ball, he or she must continue to play the second ball.

13. If you decide that a ball is unplayable (perhaps because it is next to a tree or rock), assess yourself a one-stroke penalty, drop the ball from a spot within two club lengths of the spot, and make certain that the ball is no nearer to the hole after it is dropped.

14. A player cannot touch the ground with the club if he or she is in a bunker or water hazard.

15. If you hit another player's ball while putting, it is a two-stroke penalty against you. So always ask the other players to mark their balls on the green.

One-Stroke Penalties

Unplayable lies are determined by the person playing the ball. That player can (1) drop the ball two club lengths away from the unplayable lie and count a one-stroke penalty, (2) return along the line of flight of the ball and drop it at any point, counting a one-stroke penalty, or (3) on a tee shot, return to the tee and hit again, while taking a penalty stroke.

Water hazard play occurs when a ball is hit into a body of water running between the tee and the hole. The hazard may be marked by yellow stakes outside of the water. If you are inside the yellow staked area or in the water, you can play the ball with no penalty, but you must not touch the club to the grass or the water before hitting the shot. If you prefer, you can take a one-stroke penalty and drop the ball anywhere back along the line of flight that the ball followed in getting to the water.

Lateral water hazard is water (pond or stream) that lies on the side of the fairway. It is marked by red stakes. You can play the ball as it lies, or take a one-stroke penalty and either drop the ball two club lengths away from the hazard (but not closer to the hole) or drop the ball along the flight path of the ball from the spot of your last shot.

Two-Stroke Penalty

Grounding the club in a hazard, such as water or sand, is a two-stroke penalty in stroke play. If you are playing match play, you lose the hole.

Summary

1. Every golfer must be familiar with the rules of the game.
2. The order of play on a hole is determined on the tee by having the low scorer from the previous hole hit first. The second lowest scorer hits second, etc. After the tee shot, the farthest person from the pin will be the next person to hit.
3. The objective of golf is to "play the ball where it lies." There are some situations, however, in which a player is allowed to move the ball away from an unnatural hazard.
4. Every swing counts, even if you miss the ball.
5. There are penalties for hitting out of bounds, losing a ball, and for other infractions of the rules of the game.

12 *Etiquette on the Course*

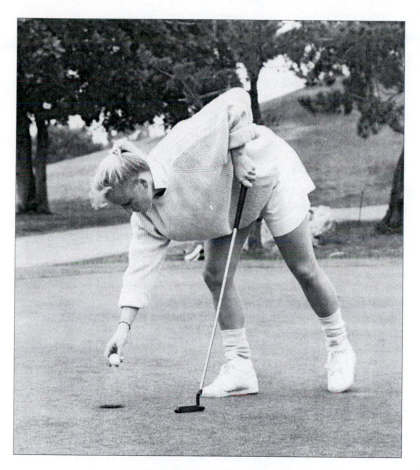

Outline

Proper golf etiquette can generally be reduced to the Golden Rule: "Do unto others as you would have them do unto you." And that's a great starting point for golf etiquette.

Respect a Golfer's Right to Silence

Allow your partners to concentrate on their shots. Do not stand in another player's line of sight. The preferred place to stand is behind the person taking a swing. If you cannot avoid standing in the periphery of the line of sight, stay motionless so that you do not inadvertently create a distraction. Do not practice your swing while another player is lining up a shot, since this can also disturb that person's concentration.

Obviously, it is important to be quiet when a person is concentrating on a practice swing or a shot. Golf requires such heavy concentration that any unexpected noises can interfere with the thinking pattern.

Etiquette on the Green

The closeness of the players on the putting green makes consideration even more important. On the putting green, always take your ball out of the cup after you have holed out. But be careful not to get in the way of a player who is lining up a putt. And don't step in the line of the putt, because your spike marks might redirect the putt.

Stand either directly behind the putter's back or directly in front some distance away. Do not stand in front of or behind the line of the putt. And be certain that your shadow doesn't fall on the player's line of putt.

On the green, the closest player to the pin should tend the pin and remove it if the person putting wants it removed. It should be placed far enough away from the line of each person's putt so that the flag does not interfere with anyone's concentration.

Be Prepared to Play Your Next Shot

Know when it is your turn to hit. On the first hole, you can flip coins or just decide who will tee off first. After the first hole, the person who has scored the best on the last hole should *have the honors* of teeing off first on the next hole. In case of a tie, the person who teed off earlier on the last hole will tee off earlier on the next tee. For example, suppose Al teed off first on the last hole, followed by Barbara, Carl, and Debra; Barbara and Debra scored with 5s, Carl with a 6, and Al with a 7. The order for the next tee would be Barbara, Debra, Carl, and Al.

After teeing off, the person farthest from the hole hits next. If the shot is very short, that person may hit again as long as he or she is still the farthest from the hole. The same holds true when everyone is on the putting green—the person farthest from the hole putts first.

Etiquette around the green

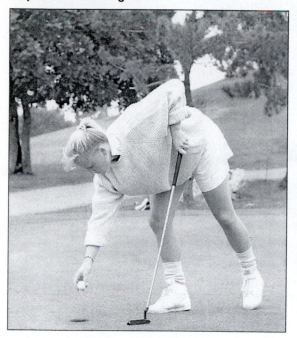

Always remove the ball from the hole before the next putter's turn

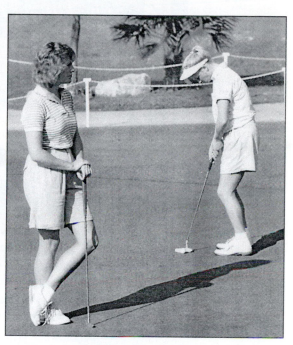

Never cast a shadow across the line of another player's putt

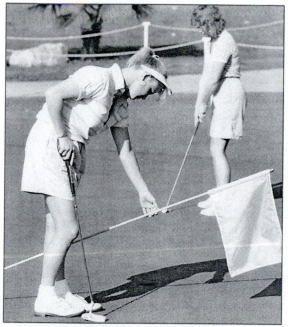

Never place the pin anywhere around the hole where it could be hit

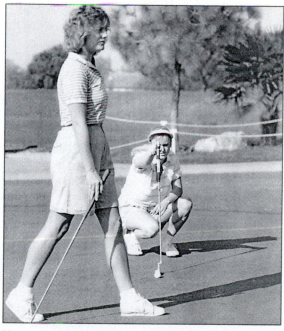

Never step in the line of another player's putt

✓ Checklist for Etiquette on the Greens

1. Mark your ball on the green so that it will not be in the line of sight of another player who is putting.
2. If your ball is closest to the hole, tend the pin, or pull it out on request and lay it down on the putting surface.
3. If you lay the pin down on the green, make sure that it is not in the line of sight of another player who is putting.
4. Do not step in the line of another player's putt between the ball and the hole.
5. Do not stand behind a player who is putting. Stay away from his or her line of sight. (The best place to stand is directly behind or face to face with the player who is putting.)
6. Line your putt up while the other players in your foursome are lining up theirs, and be ready to putt when it is your turn.
7. Do not move or talk while another player is putting
8. Move your ball marker if it is in the line of another player's putt.
9. Take your ball out of the hole after you have completed your putt.
10. When you are waiting for another player to putt, make certain that your shadow does not fall across the ball, the hole, or the line of the other player's putt.
11. Do not leave the green until all of the members of your foursome have putted out.
12. Repair all ball marks on the green.
13. When you are tending the pin, make certain that your shadow does not fall across the hole or across the line of the putt.

Speed of Play

Keep the play speeded up. If you are playing slower than the group that is following you, you should let them go ahead, or *play through*—as long as the group playing ahead of you is far ahead of you. This situation often occurs when you are in a foursome, and only two players are following you.

On par-3 holes, once you are on the green, if you see that the group behind is ready to tee off wave them on with your hand then stand behind the green until they have all hit. Then putt out.

Speeding up play is important. You should always know where everyone's balls have landed. Help your partners by watching their shots and telling them where their balls have landed. That way, if a ball is lost, you will have a better idea where to help your partner look for it.

Always be ready to hit when it is your turn. Choose your club and select your target ahead of time so that you will be ready to hit as soon as possible when it is your turn. Never take more than one practice swing when it is your shot. Then, when you address the ball, don't dally over it; just set your concentration and swing.

On par-3s, wave up the group behind you on the tee if they are ready

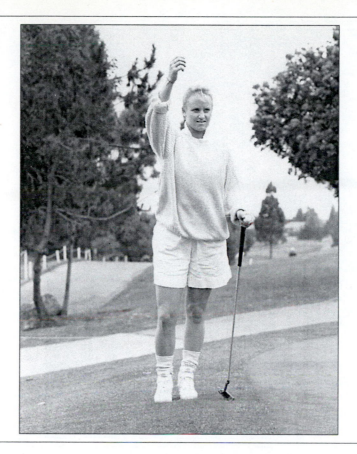

When you have finished a hole, mark your score on the card after you have left the green. There are probably others waiting to hit to the green, so get moving as quickly as possible.

 Checklist for Allowing a Group to Play Through

1. If you are far behind the group ahead of you, and the group behind you is playing more quickly than your group. allow the following group to play through.
2. If you are holding up play by looking for a lost ball, allow the following group to play through.
3. When allowing a group to play through, it is faster to let them play through on a 3-par hole rather than on a long hole.
4. When allowing a group to play through on a 3-par, mark your balls and wave the group up. When they leave the green, putt out. Then let them tee off ahead of you on the next hole.

After a full shot in the rough or fairway, replace your divot

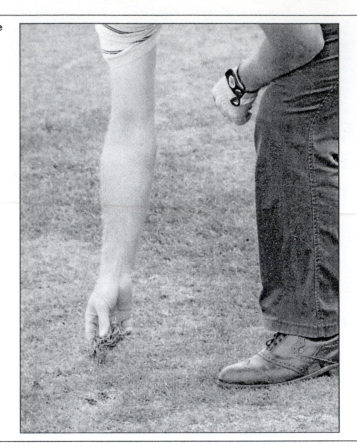

Keep the Course in Shape

Always replace your divots and tamp them down with your shoe. When you have walked in a sand trap, always rake your tracks as you leave so another player's ball won't land in your shoeprint.

On the putting green, repair any ball depressions with a green-repair tool or a tee by pushing it under the depression and lifting it back to ground level. Then tamp it down with your putter blade so that other players' putts won't be deflected by your depression mark.

The greens are such important parts of the course that special care should be taken near them. Your clubs should never be placed on the green. And, of course, your cart should be kept at a distance from the green and parked behind it—on the cart path.

If you notice some damage on a fairway, green, or bunker, repair it even if you did not cause it (as long as repairing it will not slow up the play).

"Fore!"

When you hear the shout "Fore!", cover your head, turn your back to the sound, and stay protected until you are certain that the ball has landed. It might not have even been coming in your direction, but it is better to be cautious than to be hit. "Fore" is also yelled when a person is in the way of a hitter. So cover up first, but then look to see if you are in somebody's way.

Summary

1. Always be considerate of other players.
2. Do not talk, move, or stand too close to a player who is addressing the ball.
3. Keep the play speeded up.
4. Keep safety in mind. Always let players ahead of you play until they are far enough away so that you can't hit them with a shot.
5. Always repair the fairways, traps, and greens—even if you were not the one who caused the damage.
6. Be careful not to damage the course with your practice swings.

13 *Practice and Warm-Up*

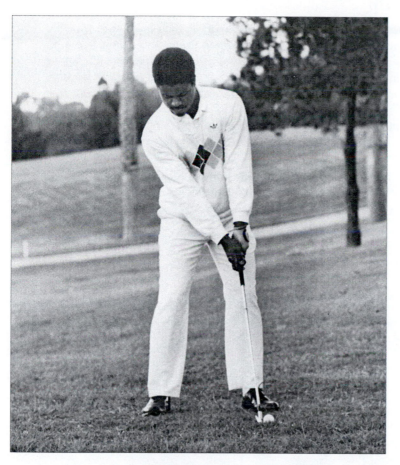

Outline

very facet of your golf game requires practice—your mental imagery, your physical coordination, and your "touch." Moreover, just as concentration is the key to a good shot on the course, it is also the key to effective practice. Remember, practice doesn't make perfect; rather, perfect practice makes perfect. Quality is more important than quantity in practicing. It is better to have shorter practice sessions more often than long ones less often.

The Warm-Up

Stretch your muscles so that they are ready to work at their maximum capacity and will not be pulled or injured when you begin to swing your clubs. If you do not stretch and warm up before you start hitting, your coordination will change slightly as your muscles become more stretched and warmed—so you will not be hitting the same way ten minutes after you started as you were on your first swings.

The next chapter will give you a complete set of stretching exercises. Some popular ones are briefly described here. Do them slowly and hold position for 20 to 30 seconds.

■ While sitting on the ground with your legs straight, touch your toes. This stretches your lower back and the back of your thighs.

Place a club behind your back and rotate your torso

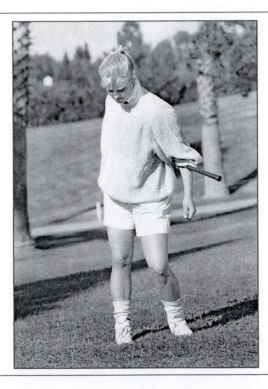

Swing the club with only the left hand on the club

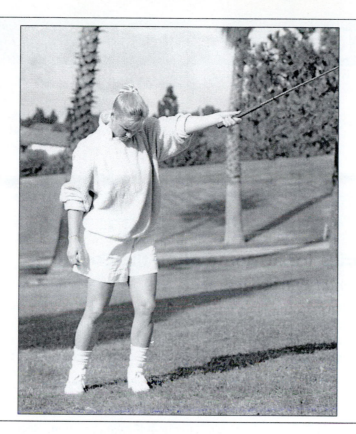

- While sitting on the ground, touch the soles of your feet together and allow your knees to move toward the floor. This stretches your groin area and prepares your legs muscles for the swing.
- With your arms extended at shoulder level, twist slowly right, then left. This prepares your very important abdominal muscles for the swing.
- Raise your arms over your head, then cross them, reaching your left arm over your head to the right and your right arm to the left. This stretches the muscles of your shoulders, your upper back, and the back of your arms.
- Put a club behind your back and just under your upper arms. Take your stance and practice your turn and weight shift. Start slowly.
- Take a club and grip it cross-handed, with your left hand on the bottom. Then take your full swing. Concentrate on your hip and shoulder turn and your weight shift.
- Hold a club in your left hand. Take your regular stance and use your regular swing—but only with your left arm and hand controlling your club.

✓   *Checklist for Warming Up*

1. Always allow yourself time to warm up. Arrive at the course a half hour or more before your tee time.
2. Stretch the muscles that you will use during your play. Then warm up your muscles by swinging one, two, or three clubs at one time. Swing slowly at first.
3. Lay a driver across the back of your shoulders and practice your hip turn before you hit any practice balls.

Drills for at Home or on the Course

Mental Practice

Mental practice will be detailed in the last chapter. Let us emphasize here the importance of mental practice and the fact that you can practice your imagery, mental and physical rehearsal, relaxation techniques, and concentration every day, since no special setting or equipment is required.

Setting the Base

To practice setting the "base" of your golf swing position, place a golf ball under the outside edge of your right foot. This will keep you from putting your weight on the outside of that foot. It will also keep your right knee from sliding to the outside and destroying your base. If you hit some balls this way, you will see that your base is solid.

Working on the Y-Shape

To practice the Y-shape of your golf-swing, bring the club back halfway through the backswing, then swing the Y-shape formed by both arms and the club. Finish by extending your left arm and holding the Y position.

Ball Alignment

Ball alignment can be checked by placing one club along your toes. Line the ball up in front of the inside of your left heel. Take your driver and lay it on the inside of your left heel and at a right angle to the other club that is touching your toes. Does the driver touch the ball? If so, it is properly aligned.

Practice maintaining the Y with half swings

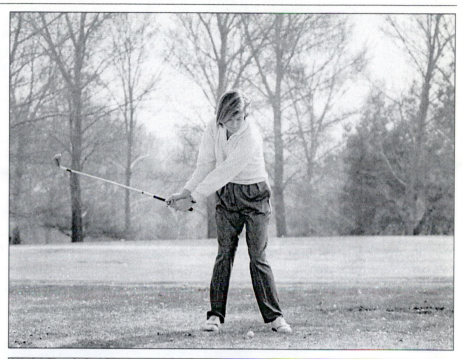

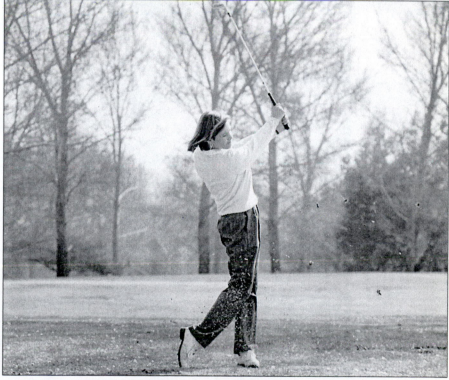

Cross-Handed Putting

Practice cross-handed putting on your living room carpet to help eliminate wrist movement in your putting stroke. Putt with your left hand lower on the club than your right.

Aiming Your Putt

Whether putting on the practice green or your living room carpet, pick a spot on the green or carpet and putt to it. Get about 3 or 4 feet back from the spot and look only at the spot, not the ball. See how close you come to the target with ten putts.

Drills on the Practice Tee

Balance

Balance can be improved by hitting iron shots with your feet together rather than from your regular stance. Take a full swing with your driver, and as you

Practice your balance by hitting iron shots with your feet together

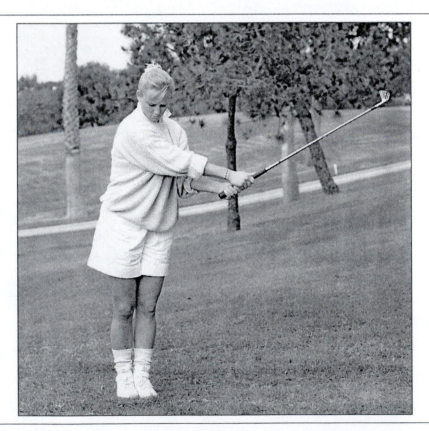

Practice taking a full swing with your driver and then lifting your right foot

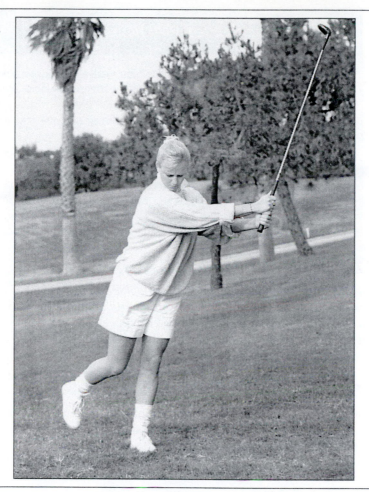

follow through, lift your right foot off the ground and balance on your left leg. Hit some drives to see if you are off balance because you have been hitting too hard.

Hitting with Your Legs

To practice "hitting with your legs" (that is, using leg strength in your swing), place the ball out in front of your left toe instead of farther back in your stance. Swing your driver and push yourself forward to the ball with your right leg. Reach out and sweep the ball off the tee with an upward swing of the clubface at contact.

✓   *Checklist for Practicing*

1. When hitting practice balls, start with your wedge and hit short pitch shots. Progressively work your way up through the irons and woods, finishing with your driver.
2. If you do not want to use every club in your bag, use either the even-numbered or the odd-numbered irons only.
3. Practice some chip shots to the practice green and sink a few putts just before moving to the first tee.
4. If you do not have time to hit practice shots before a match, make certain that you do the stretching exercises and swing a club before teeing off.

Decide on Your Practice Plan

Ask yourself the following questions: Do you want to use all of your clubs from wedge to driver? Do you want to concentrate on mid-irons? Do you want to concentrate on your weight shift and leg power? Do you want to work on a special type of shot, such as an intentional slice or hook?

Special Shots

If you are an advanced player, you might want to develop an arsenal of varied trajectories. To hit over, under, or around trees or other objects, you need to develop arcs that are not normal for a standard swing.

Intentional Hook

An intentional hook can be developed by using any or all of the following adjustments to your stance and swing:

- Close your stance (left foot forward).
- Turn your hands to the right, or set up with your clubface closed.
- Swing the club back more to the inside than you normally do.

Intentional Slice

An intentional slice can be developed by any or all of the following adjustments to your stance and swing:

- Open your stance (left foot back).
- Turn your hands to the left, or open your clubface on address.
- Swing your club back more to the outside of your normal swing.

The intentional hook versus the intentional slice

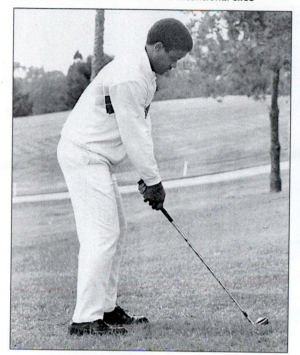

Close your stance for the hook

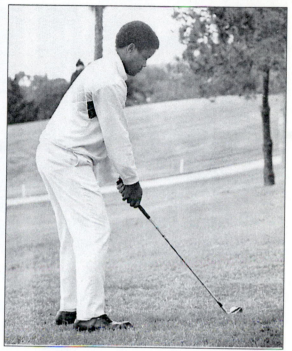

Open your stance for the slice

Intentional High Ball

An intentional high ball can be hit by making the following adjustments:

- Play the ball closer to your target than normal (more to the left for right-handers).
- Set up with your hands even with or slightly behind the ball.
- Open the clubface slightly.
- Set up with more weight on your rear foot (the right foot for right-handers), and keep your head and body slightly behind the ball when you are swinging forward.

Intentional Low Ball

An intentional low ball is often required when hitting from under the trees. To accomplish this shot:

- Play the ball back in your stance (closer to the right foot for right-handers).
- Set up with your hands ahead of the ball when addressing it.
- Close the clubface slightly.
- Hit down and through the ball. Use less than normal wrist action.

The intentional high ball versus the intentional low ball

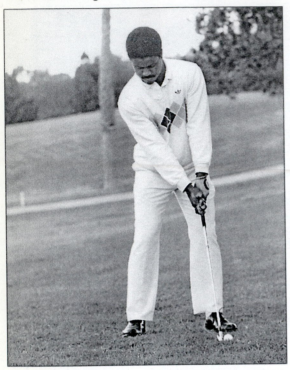 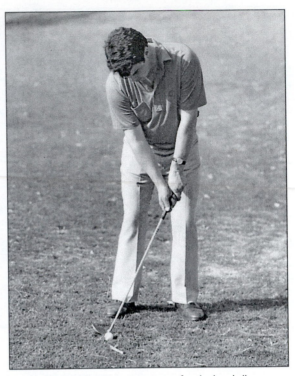

Move the ball forward in your stance for the high ball   Move the ball backward in your stance for the low ball

Summary

1. To practice or play efficiently, and to avoid injury, you must warm up properly.

2. It is very important to stretch the muscles that you will use in your golf game.

3. You can practice mentally as well as physically.

4. Many of the skills of golf can be practiced at home; others are best practiced at the practice tee—the driving range.

5. Always have a plan for your practice.

6. Your objective should be *perfect* practice, not merely practice. So concentrate as much while practicing as you would do on the course.

14 *Improving Your Game Through Strength and Flexibility*

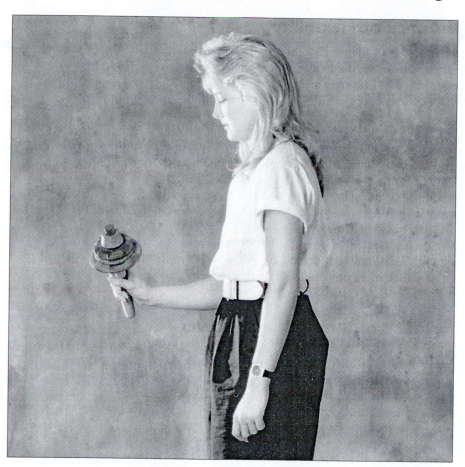

Outline

The average golfer works with an inefficient body, neither as strong nor as flexible as it needs to be for an adequate performance. Yet, everyone can increase flexibility and strength. For the average golfer who has not done flexibility or strength exercises before, the improvement is dramatic once such exercises are begun. For the well-conditioned athlete, improvement is slower, but it will nevertheless occur. Players at every level will benefit from these exercises.

Importance of Flexibility

A more flexible body allows us to bring the club back farther for a more complete swing. Obviously, the longer a force can be applied to an object, the greater its speed. So a longer swing can generate more clubhead speed at impact. Of course, a longer swing is of no benefit if the club cannot be controlled.

In addition to making our swing more powerful, correct stretching exercises make our muscles and connective tissues more capable of delivering an efficient and accurate swing. Moreover, properly conditioned muscles reduce the possibility of injuries.

Correctly done, flexibility exercises stretch the connective tissues (such as tendons and ligaments), allowing us to swing in a more complete arc. The same exercises also help tense muscles relax.

If you are flexible, you will be able to turn your body and arms farther back. You will be able to start your downward swing with more power—and with less effort. You will be more powerful while being more relaxed.

Importance of Strength and Power

Strength occurs when you are able to make more muscle fibers contract at the same time. Muscle fibers are very small—about the size of a human hair. Each fiber either contracts fully or not at all. For example, when you lift a glass of water to your mouth, some of the muscle fibers in your biceps muscle will contract completely, but many will stay relaxed.

As you gain strength, you will be able to make more muscle fibers contract at one time. If you can contract 200 fibers in a certain muscle at one time before starting your strength program, you might eventually be able to contract 250, 300, or even 500 at one time. This ability to make more muscle fibers work at the same time is what we call strength.

In most athletic events, we need more than strength—we need power. Power is a combination of speed and strength. If you will work on gaining strength while continuing to practice your golf swing, you should develop effective power. You will also become more resistant to injury.

Exercises for Flexibility

Stretching should be done slowly, and each stretch should be held for 20 to 30 seconds. For best results, stretching should be done daily and after you are warmed up, and each stretch should be repeated six times. But even doing these exercises once every other day will help.

The following exercises are ranked according to their importance. So if you can't do them all, do what you can, starting from the first ones on the list. And if you don't have time to do them each six times, just do them once. Anything is better than nothing.

1. *Full abdominal twist:* Perhaps the most important area in which to gain flexibility is in the abdominal muscles and tendons. Full rotation is the key to a powerful golf swing. It is impossible to rotate and coil your body if you do not have a full range of motion.

   For the full abdominal twist, face away from a wall with your feet about 18 inches apart. Turn toward the wall, putting both of your hands on the wall. This allows for a more complete backswing and follow-through. Be sure to do it to each side.

2. *Triceps stretch:* The next most important area for flexibility is the shoulder girdle. If you can lift your left arm higher (as a right-handed golfer), you increase your arc and can thus apply power to your clubhead for a longer

Full abdominal twist

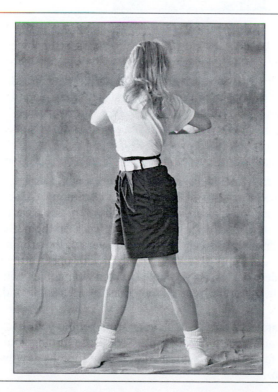

Triceps stretch

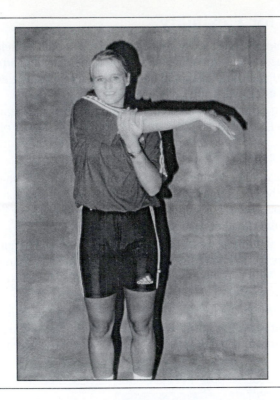

distance. In addition, by stretching the muscles in the lower part of your left shoulder, you will generate more power—with less effort.

For the triceps stretch, assuming that you are right-handed, push your left arm up next to your right chest with your right arm. Your left arm should be in the same postion as it will be during your backswing. This exercise will stretch the triceps muscle and allow you to reach higher in your swing. This will then allow you to apply speed to the clubhead for a longer distance and therefore deliver more power. Repeat with the other arm.

3. *Rotator cuff stretch:* Golfers and other athletes who throw or hit in their sports use some seldom heard of muscles commonly called *rotator cuff muscles.* These muscles are deep under the skin. Since they can't be shown off at the beach, most body builders don't work on them. But golfers must work on them because they are prime movers of the arm in the golf swing. Note that at the top of your swing, both of your upper arms have rotated in their shoulder sockets. As you unleash your swing, they will rotate in the other direction. For this reason, they must be as flexible and as strong as possible.

For the rotator cuff stretch, with your arms behind your back and with your hands at waist level, pull your arms back while turning your thumbs upward as far as they can go; then turn your thumbs downward as far as they can go.

Neck stretch and twists

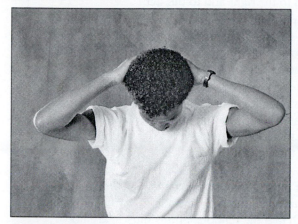

Push your head forward

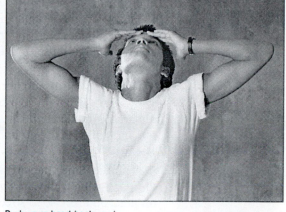

Push your head backward

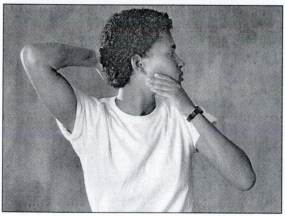

Pull your head to the left side

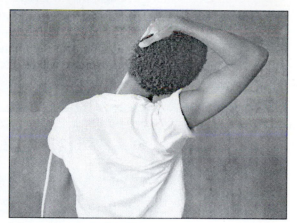

Pull your head to the right side

Another rotator cuff stretch can be done as follows: While sitting or standing, stretch both arms out to your side (at a 90-degree angle to the side of your body). Now bend your elbows to a 90-degree angle and allow the forearm to move backward so that your upper arm is turning in the shoulder joint. You should feel the stretch in the front of your shoulders.

4. *Side stretch:* Another abdominal stretching exercise is the side stretch, since it is so important to be able to use your trunk muscles through a full range of motion. With your feet about 2 feet apart, bend sideways. This increases the flexibility in the side area of your abdominal muscles.

5. *Neck stretch and twists:* Because in the golf swing we rotate our bodies while our heads remain relatively motionless, we must have great flexibility in our necks. Without sufficient flexibility, our heads will move with our shoulders as we coil in our backswings.

For neck stretches and twists, push your head forward, backward and to each side; then turn your head to the right and to the left.

6. *Groin stretch:* We start our swings with our legs. The primary movers are the muscles in the groin area. For the groin stretch, spread your legs 3 to 4 feet apart. Squat down and move your weight over your right leg. This will stretch the groin muscles of the left leg. Hold the stretch. Now stretch the other leg.

7. *Trunk stretch:* This is another stretch for your abdominals as well as your lower back. Lie flat on your back, bend your left knee, then roll your hips so that your left knee touches the floor to the right of your right leg. Keep your shoulders on the ground throughout the exercise. Repeat with right knee bent.

8. *"Lats" stretch:* Since the largest muscle that is stretched when you are doing your backswing is the *latissimus dorsi* (the large muscle of the upper back), you need an exercise to stretch it. If the tendons of this muscle are not long enough, they will reduce your backswing.

For the "lats" stretch, reach your arms over your head and cross them. Pull your right elbow toward your neck with your left hand. Repeat, pulling your left elbow with your right hand. You will feel the stretch under your shoulders. This exercise will also stretch your rotator cuff.

Groin stretch

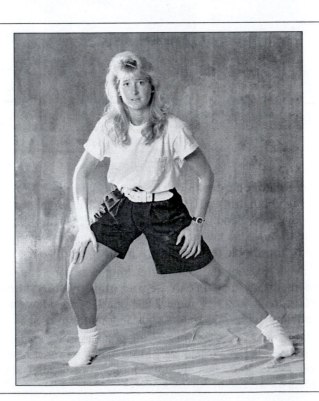

The "lats" stretch

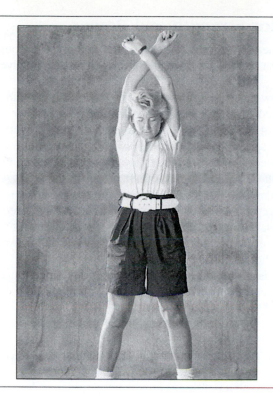

✓ *Checklist for Stretching*

1. Hold every stretch for 20 to 30 seconds.
2. Stretch your abdominals by the full sideways twist to each side, not by bending backward.
3. Stretch and twist the neck.
4. Stretch your "lats" (latissimus dorsi muscles) by crossing your arms over your head.
5. Stretch your rotator cuff muscles.
6. Stretch your groin muscles.
7. Stretch your triceps.

Exercises for Strength and Power

There is a best method for stretching each joint and muscle group in the body, and there is a best method for strengthening each muscle involved in the swing.

Strength is how much weight you can lift. Power is a combination of strength and speed. Most golf movements require power rather than brute strength. You must, however, work to increase both your power and strength. Some gyms have special machines for developing power; but even if you don't have access to special machines, your strength work, when combined with the speed of your golf swing, will increase your power in the swing.

For maximum results, you should exhaust the muscle in six repetitions. Do three sets of six repetitions each. Give your muscles two or three minutes to rest between sets. During this rest period, you can do exercises for other muscles. If you can only do one set each workout, you will still increase your strength, though not as quickly.

Strength exercises should be done every other day, since muscles take about 48 hours to recover from an effective workout. You might do half of the exercises one day and the other half the next day.

But remember, any workout will help you. If you exercise only once a week, that will help.

You strengthen a muscle by making it work against resistance. Most people use iron weights. Many weight lifters today use machines of various sorts, but you can also use manual resistance in which you use your hands or those of a partner to provide the resistance.

The following exercises are listed in order of importance, so if you don't have time to do all of them, start with the first ones and do what you can. You will still be able to make a measurable improvement in your game.

1. *Twisting sit-ups:* As previously emphasized, the abdominal muscles are critical in developing power in the golf swing. Here is an exercise that emphasizes the twisting action in the swing.

   For twisting sit-ups, with knees bent and your hands on your chest, curl up and touch your left elbow to your right knee and return to the starting position. Repeat, touching your right elbow to your left knee. As you get stronger, you can add weight by holding weight plates, dumbbells, or books on your chest.

2. *Wrist-strength exercises:* The wrist is the final area of the body that develops power at impact. If the wrists are strong, they add to that power. If they are weak, they actually bend backward at impact and cannot transmit the power that the rest of the body has developed. Most people have weak wrists. Consequently, strengthening them is of critical importance in developing a powerful golf swing.

   For these wrist-strength exercises, use a partially weighted dumbbell (weight on only one end). For maximum strength, the weight should be sufficiently heavy so that you can exhaust your muscles in six to ten repetitions. However, any heavy resistance will help your wrist power.

Twisting sit-up

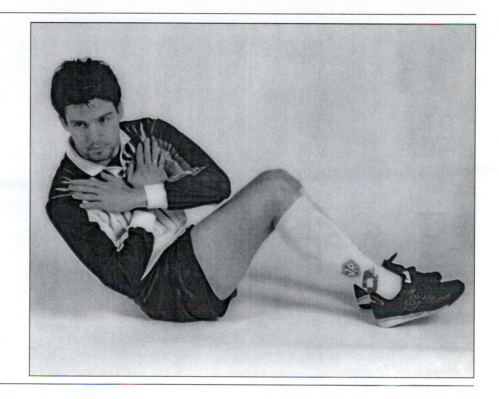

Hold the weight with the weighted end toward the little finger side of your hand. Twist the wrist back to an upright position. This strengthens the muscles that uncoil the hands at impact. This exercise can be done standing or sitting.

If you are supplying your own resistance, just hold the top of your right hand in your left palm. Bend your right hand backward. Give it resistance. Then put your left palm in your right palm and bend your right wrist upward. Do this six times, then change hands.

You don't have to use weights to strengthen your wrist. Just as you can use one of your hands to give yourself resistance, you can also use a broom. To develop the back of your wrist, hold the broom with your palm down, and move the broom with your wrist extending upward. This is particularly helpful for the leading arm in your swing (the left forearm for right-handers). To develop the inside part of your forearm, hold the broomstick with your palm up. This is particularly helpful for the right forearm for right-handed golfers.

The back of the forearm is another underused muscle. The muscles in the back of the left forearm (for right-handers) help to straighten the wrists at impact with the ball. Back-of-forearm strength is best developed by doing reverse wrist curls. Take a weight, straddle a bench, and with the palm facing down, raise the weight.

Wrist-strength exercise with dumbbell

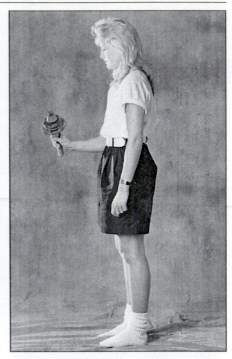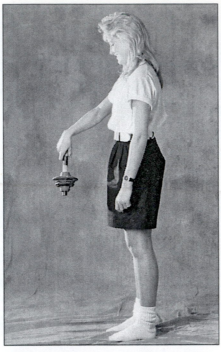

Use a partially weighted dumbbell

Twist wrist back to upright position

Wrist-strength exercise with manual resistance

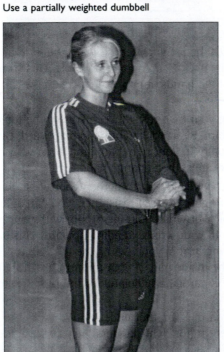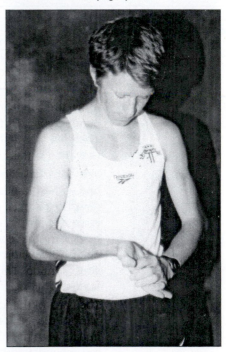

Bend wrist downward against resistance

Bend wrist upward against resistance

Wrist-strength exercise with broomstick

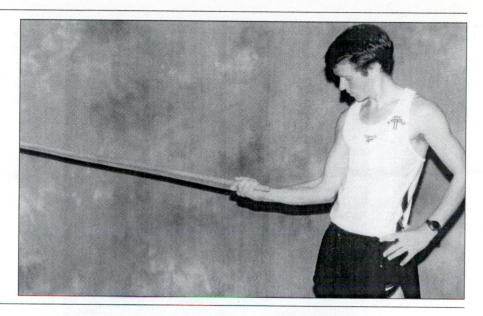

If you are supplying your own resistance, just bend one hand forward at the wrist, then put your other hand on the back of the hand to be exercised. Raise that hand upward as far as possible. Repeat six times, and then change hands.

Back-of-forearm strength exercise with manual resistance

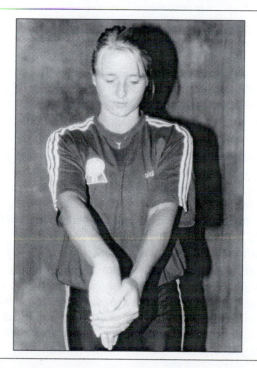

Shoulder extension and twist

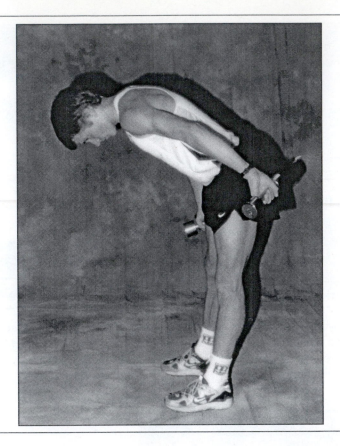

The following twisting exercise strengthens muscles that come into play at the impact of the clubhead with the ball. With the resistance of one hand on the thumb side of the other hand and your forearm parallel to the ground, twist the hand to one side then the other, giving resistance in both directions.

3. *Arm pull:* We start the downward pull of our arms with the muscles in the left shoulder and upper left arm. For the arm pull exercise, it is best to have a "lat" machine—this machine has an overhead pulley that allows you to pull the resistance down. Standing sideways to the machine, grip the pulley cable (not the handle) the same way you would grip the club (the palm of your hand pointing backward), then pull the cable across your body just as you would do in a golf swing. Right-handers do it with the left arm and left-handers with the right arm.

   This exercise can also be done using surgical rubber bands (available at most pharmacies). Anchor one end of the rubber high on a wall, or tie a knot on one end, put that end on the top of a door, and close the door, squeezing the rubber between the top of the door and the door jamb. Tie another knot in the other end and grip the rubber above the knot, then pull down as you would on a "lat" machine (explained above).

Internal rotator cuff rotation

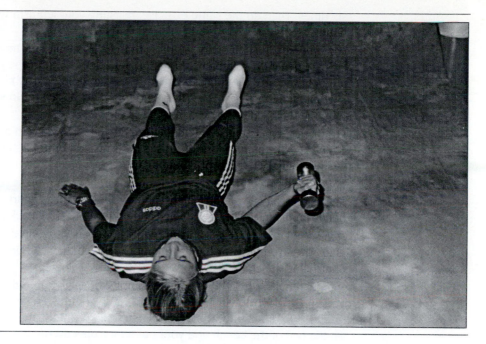

To supply your own resistance, put your right hand on your left elbow (for right-handers), pull your left arm down through the impact area, and continue into the follow-through. It is better if you can do this exercise with a partner supplying the resistance, because a partner can give you more resistance.

4. *Rotator cuff rotation:* As previously mentioned, the rotator cuff muscles are very important in golf. The arms rotate in their shoulder-joint sockets throughout the backswing, then they rotate the other way during the downswing and follow-through. They must be strong both for swing power and to avoid injury.

   While bending forward with dumbbells (or books or bricks) in your hands, lift them backward to shoulder height while twisting your palms inward (thumbs down).

   For external rotator cuff rotation, lie on your right side with a dumbbell in your left hand and with your elbow bent at 90 degrees. Then lift the weight until your forearm is straight up. Repeat on the other side.

   For internal rotation, lie on your back, dumbbell in hand and elbow bent at 90 degrees, and lift the dumbbell to the straight-up position (with your elbow still on the ground).

   If you are supplying your own resistance, bend your right forearm to 90 degrees at the elbow. Hold the back of your right hand with your left hand, and rotate your right forearm outward. Then put your left hand in the palm of your right, and twist your right arm back in as far as it will go. Repeat six times. Then do the same exercise, resisting your left arm with your right hand.

5. *Leg squeeze:* The golf swing starts with the legs. While our major leg muscles are generally relatively strong, the muscles that start the golf swing are not. They are the muscles that one uses in doing a frog kick while swimming the breast stroke. It is therefore a good idea to do some special work on these underworked muscles.

   For the leg squeeze, use an adductor machine or work with a partner. Squeeze your thighs together (this is the same action that starts your golf swing); then try to separate them against resistance.

   If you are supplying your own resistance, sit on a chair, press your hands against the outside of your thighs, and move your knees apart. Then put your hands on the inside of your thighs, and bring your knees back together.

6. *Hand-strength exercises:* Hand strength is obviously essential in holding the club. The stronger your hands, the more relaxed they can be while still controlling the club.

   Hand strength is best developed by simply squeezing an old tennis ball. If you prefer to work with weights, you can do some wrist curls. The simplest way is to take a dumbbell or barbell, straddle a bench, and with your wrist on the end of the bench and your palm face up, curl the weight up toward your forearm.

7. *Triceps-strength exercise:* The triceps muscle is involved in the arm action that brings the club downward toward the ball. Some of the preceding exercises work the triceps in combination with other muscles, but here is an exercise for just the triceps:

   With a dumbbell or book in one hand, straighten that arm upward. Take your other hand and place it on the elbow of the arm carrying the weight. Let the dumbbell come down behind your back by bending your elbow; then straighten your arm. Hold the elbow of the lifting arm so that the upper part of your arm is always straight. Repeat the exercise with the other arm.

   If you are supplying your own resistance, just bend your left arm at the elbow as far up as it will go, then put your right hand on your left wrist and push against your hand until your left arm is straight. Repeat six times, and then exercise the other arm.

Finding Time to Exercise

Although some golfers have nearly unlimited time to work on their golf games and to stay fit by working out at gyms, many of us have very busy schedules. Still, if you want to improve your game, you must take time in that busy schedule for exercise. Each exercise takes only a few seconds, and since you can use yourself for the resistance, you can work out anywhere.

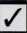 **Checklist for Developing Strength for Golf**

1. Do the twisting sit-ups.
2. Strengthen the wrist with the several exercises designed for wrist strength.
3. Develop strength in your "lats" muscle, which is a primary mover in the downward pull of the club.
4. Do the rotator cuff exercises. This is an important muscle group that is usually neglected by golfers in their training.
5. Do thigh-squeezing exercises.
6. Strengthen the hand muscles so that they can control the club even though they are not gripping it tightly.
7. Strengthen the back of your forearm, especially the target arm (left forearm for right-handed golfers).
8. Strengthen the triceps muscle (back of the arm) so that it can add power on the downward swing as you uncoil your arms.

It takes less than ten minutes to do each of the strength exercises six times, using yourself as the resistance. In two to five more minutes, you can do each of the stretching exercises at least once. So if you alternate stretching and strength exercises daily, you can gain substantial benefits in less than five minutes a day. Those five minutes will benefit you more than any other five minutes you can spend practicing the game of golf.

Many of these exercises can be done in the classroom, the office, while driving, or while relaxing at home in front of the TV. They don't have to take up much time. Why don't you give them a try?

Summary

1. Every participant in a sport can profit from increased strength and flexibility.
2. Flexibility exercises will allow a golfer to be able to swing the club through a greater range of motion and to develop more power (because the clubhead will travel farther through the swing).
3. In the golf swing, you can be only as strong as the weakest link in your swing. For that reason, you must work on every aspect of your swing—legs, abdominals, shoulders, arms, and wrists.

15 Improving Your Game with the Power of Your Mind

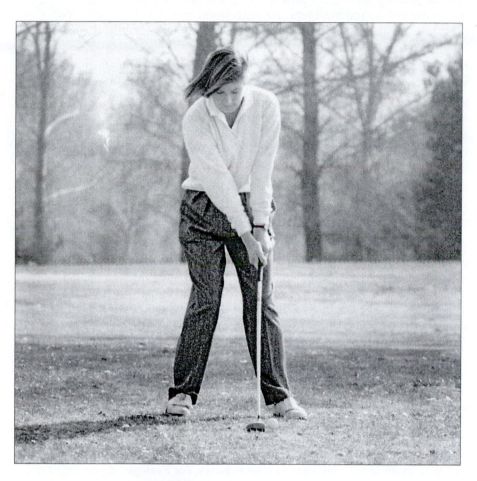

Outline

An old golf adage states that "the toughest six inches on the golf course are between your ears." Instead of blaming your clubs, the course, or the weather when you don't play well, start by concentrating on the key to the game—your mind. Your performance will improve if you learn how to focus your mind on a task, how to relax, and how to control your mind.

After you have perfected your basic swing, you can begin to practice mentally in the following ways:

1. *Imagine* yourself making the perfect swing. It is not enough to imagine your basic swing. You must rehearse each wood, iron, and your putt. You must also imagine the types of shots and putts you will probably be making on the next course you will play.

2. Next you will want to physically *rehearse* your shots. There are effective ways to physically and mentally rehearse the shots you expect to make.

3. When on the course, you will need to *relax* to be able to reduce your tension and anxiety. You will want to be able to totally relax before every shot, since tension will make your muscles less able to work effectively.

4. Once you are relaxed and ready, you must *concentrate* on just one single thing as you swing.

Mental Imagery and Rehearsal

Many athletes have mentally practiced their events prior to their performances. A high jumper will imagine going through the jump prior to making the attempt at the bar. A diver will always imagine spinning and twisting through the next dive. The high jumper needs to imagine only one type of jumping action. The diver must have at least ten dives in his or her repertoire, so a number of different actions must be imagined. But golf is more complex even than diving and thus provides more opportunity for using this highly successful technique of *mental imagery* to improve our performance.

Mental imagery is not daydreaming. It is practice. Mental imagery is the technique that programs your mind to make your body respond as it has been programmed. And learning how to do it is essential if you are to maximize your potential as a golfer.

Mental practice has a real physical dimension to it: you are actually training your muscles as you think about making a shot. When you mentally visualize moving, your brain sends messages to your muscles. For example, if you are thinking about taking the club back with your left arm, the muscles in the front of your left arm will tense as you think about it. They won't contract as much as they will when you are executing the actual swing, but they will be learning how you want them to work when you are ready to take your backswing.

Some athletes like to envision themselves going through the motions. They like to see themselves from the outside. Some like to imagine the feeling of doing the action. They like to view themselves from the inside. So imagery can be viewed from either the outside or the inside—with you as the spectator or as the participant. Both ways have their uses.

If you want to practice your swing, you might start from the outside. Jack Nicklaus called this "going to the movies." The question is, who will star in the movie? If you are not sure about how to swing a club, you might start with one of the excellent videotapes available on golf. Just pop a tape into your VCR, and let the pro on the tape become the star of your mental practice.

Next you can substitute yourself in the movie. See yourself making the perfect swing. Do you see your weight shift? Do you see your slow take-away? Do you see yourself pausing at the top of the swing? Do you see the power in your legs as they start the swing? Do you see your head down? Do you see your follow-through? We recommend ten minutes each day doing this type of imagery.

Once you have "seen" yourself from the outside, you can begin to do your imagery from the inside and "feel" your swing. Are you taking the club back slow and low? Do you feel your wrists cock? Can you feel the power in your legs as you begin your smooth swing? Do you feel your shoulders rotating around your head? Do you see the impact of the clubhead with the ball? Do you feel your full follow-through?

"Watch" yourself from the front, the rear, from each side, and the top. Then get inside yourself. How does it feel to swing your driver? How about your 5-iron? What about a 50-foot chip shot?

You can use this mental imagery while sitting or lying down, but it is more effective if you mentally rehearse while you are in your stance. When imagining yourself making your swing, make certain that it is a perfect swing. Never mentally practice a mistake. Remember, you are preparing yourself for the perfect execution of a golf shot, not an imperfect one.

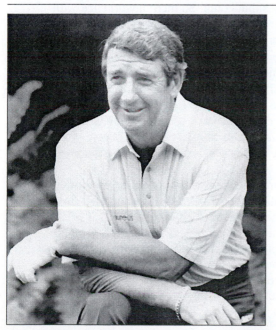

J. C. Says:

"Mental imagery can help you think positively rather than negatively. Many golfers are so conscious of the water or bunker that they hit it right into the trouble. They should be thinking positively of where they want to hit it, not where they don't want to hit. You should have the mental image of exactly where you want the ball to go. It's amazing how often you will hit it where your mind's eye sees it going."

From the Part to the Whole

If you like, particularly if you are a beginner, feel free to mentally practice only a part of the swing. Mentally feel your grip and start your backswing. Or perhaps you want to start at the top of the swing and feel the power of your legs beginning your movement. You may also want to rehearse in slow motion so that you can check every part of your swing.

Eventually you should practice the whole swing rather than just the parts. Your swing time should speed up until it is done in "real" time, that is, the swing in your mind should be just as fast, or just as slow, as it will be on the course.

What to Mentally Practice

What is it that you need most? Ask your partners or your pro to help you analyze your game. What areas appear to be the most in need of your attention? How do you handle the rough? What about an uphill lie? Does that 3-par hole over the water cause you anxiety? Does it bother you when a partner makes fun of you?

You can also rehearse handling your own self-criticism. Imagine yourself making a poor shot and then criticizing yourself. Now imagine that same poor shot, but with you focusing only on your next shot and completely forgetting about the muffed shot.

You don't want to limit your mental rehearsal to just your tee shots. While we would all like to look good when our partners are watching, we all know that the shots near the pin are the ones that count. So mentally practice with your wedge from 100 yards out, from 95, from 30. Practice with the pin near you, with the pin away. Imagine the green sloping toward you, and away from you. If you know the course, mentally practice from each part of every fairway.

As you advance in your ability to mentally rehearse your game, mentally play one hole each day. Rehearse each shot ten times. Imagine your drive. Practice your approach shots. Practice getting out of a trap or over the water. How far back should you take your wedge if you are 50 yards away with the green sloping away, the pin set deep, and with heavy rough just beyond the green? Imagine a perfect putt. See the ball drop from 50 feet out. Remember, this is practice—not daydreaming.

Before hitting, visualize and concentrate on the fundamental technique of the shot that you want to hit. Think about the proper foot position, your backswing, stroke, and follow-through. Then rehearse them mentally.

As you are approaching the tee, start to visualize your tee shot. See where the trouble is and think about how you will hit it to a spot away from that trouble. Which club will make the shot you want? Do you want to lay up short of trouble? Do you want to fade away from trouble? Which club will allow you to play within yourself and make the shot in which you have confidence? Now feel yourself make the shot. Feel your body make a complete swing and see the ball going where you want it to go.

Don't, however, stand too long over the ball. This will only create more tension. Visualize your shot, then get on with the game.

When and Where to Mentally Practice

Start your imagery sessions in a relaxed non-stressful environment. Just close your eyes and begin. As you become more proficient, open your eyes, because you will have your eyes open on the course.

Once you learn to mentally rehearse, you can take that skill anywhere. Use it on the practice tee. Use it while stopped in traffic. Use it in the classroom while waiting for your class to begin or at the office during a lull in activity. And definitely use it before making any shot on the course. Effective imagery can be done anywhere, at any time. You are limited only by your imagination.

Where appropriate, you can follow your mental rehearsal of your shot with a physical rehearsal. Everyone takes a practice swing before hitting a drive. This is an example of physical rehearsal or "simulation." But there are more things that you can practice physically.

You can physically rehearse some things that bother you. *For example*: Does it seem to inhibit your swing if you are wearing a sweater or jacket? If so, you can practice with two jackets. Then when you get into competition, the one jacket will not be noticed.

What are your problems? Uphill lies, downhill lies, bunker shots, partners' comments, can all be simulated and can aid you in reducing the anxiety that they cause.

What You Should Expect from Effective Mental Rehearsing

Obviously, you expect to improve your game with effective imagery, but it's unrealistic to expect everything to fall into place the first time on the course. If you are mentally changing a part of your swing, it may take some time before that part of the swing becomes part of the "groove." And sometimes a change in one part of the swing will affect the timing of the whole swing. So it may take a while for your body to absorb the change that your mind has made.

If you have been practicing correctly with your mind, some changes may reflect immediately in your score. If you know that you should bring the club back to a certain point to chip 40 yards and you practice that, it will reflect immediately on your game. Bring the correct information from the practice tee and your teacher into your mind so that you can practice effectively. The more specific your information, the better you can mentally rehearse. And the better your mental rehearsal, the more likely it will be quickly assimilated into your game.

Checklist for Mental Imagery

1. Decide on which type of shot or which part of a swing you want to mentally practice.
2. Either use a videotape of a professional performing the swing, or imagine watching yourself make a perfect swing.
3. Next, imagine yourself making the swing, "feeling" it in your mind.

Relaxation

Every athletic event requires the ability to relax—sometimes prior to the action, such as when a defensive lineman rests before the ball is snapped, and sometimes during the action, as when a marathon runner settles into a rhythm during a race, or when a golfer executes a short chip shot. When muscles are relaxed, they are better able to work effectively.

This principle applies to the golf swing in the following way. If you are relaxed, you can take the club farther back. This will stretch the muscles that begin the downswing, and you will have more power.

Your mind and body work together, so your mind determines whether your body will be tense. For example, when you are driving on a crowded highway, you may anxiously be looking for cars following too closely or for an opening to change lanes. This mental anxiety might produce muscle tension in your upper shoulders and neck. This might result in a headache. Your blood pressure might rise. Your stomach might secrete excess acid. You might perspire. All these physical reactions would reflect the state of your mind.

As an athlete you must be able to control your *arousal state*—that is, being relaxed or aroused when you want to be. Golfers want to be relaxed just about all the time. Some arousal is needed during the swing. A little arousal is needed during a putt. But the golfer never requires the amount of arousal that is needed by an offensive lineman making a block or by a shot-putter driving across the ring.

Techniques of Relaxation

Several years ago, Dr. Herbert Benson, a Harvard University cardiologist, developed an easy way to learn to relax, called *relaxation response*. A description follows:

Find a quiet place. Sit in a chair. Loosen your clothing. Close your eyes. Breathe deeply. And don't think.

It is the "not thinking" that is the key. If you can "not think," your mind will forget about its anxieties and become calm—and your body will relax. In order

---

✓ *Checklist for Relaxation*

1. Sit comfortably and loosen your shoes and clothing.
2. Close your eyes and breathe deeply.
3. Block out your conscious thoughts by either concentrating on your breathing, thinking "breath in, breathe out," or saying an unexciting word with each breath.

---

to eliminate thinking, you must concentrate on something that will not excite your mind and let it wander. If, as you breathe, you think "money, money, money," your mind will be active. But if you think of an unexciting word, or if you silently repeat "breathe in, breathe out" with each breath, you will be able to block out the thoughts that make you tense.

Those who want the physical benefits (such as lowered blood pressure) from Benson's relaxation response should practice it for 15 to 20 minutes once or twice a day. If you just want to learn to relax for your golf game, five minutes a day should be sufficient.

Once you learn what it feels like to relax, you will be able to do it in just three breaths. Simply think "inhale . . . exhale . . . inhale . . . exhale . . . inhale . . . exhale," and you will become relaxed. Your mind can't think of two things at the same time. So anxiety and worry will disappear if you are totally involved in "not thinking" while you are breathing deeply.

Relaxing Before Taking Your Shot

Once you have chosen your club, take your three deep breaths slowly, repeating "inhale . . . exhale." Then do the mental rehearsal for your shot—that is, go through your swing mentally. Then rehearse it physically. Address the ball. Take three more deep breaths. Now make your shot.

Concentration

The final stage of preparing for an action in sports is concentration. By concentrating on a target or perhaps a muscle, an athlete can protect his or her mind from distractions.

Often it is the clutter of thoughts in a person's mind that inhibits a maximum effort. Whether it is an unhappy home life, a mid-term test, or the noise of the crowd—a person cannot make his or her best golf shot unless the mind is concentrating on golf.

On the practice tee, you might concentrate on each sector of your swing: taking the club back slowly, starting the swing with your legs, keeping your left arm straight, or finishing the stroke with a full follow-through. But you can concentrate on only one at a time. When the sector of the swing you want to improve becomes automatic, you can move to the next sector. Once the swing becomes grooved, you will need to concentrate only on the ball.

Strangely, the ball is often the major distraction to learning to swing. Beginners sometimes put so much effort into hitting the ball that they can't concentrate on improving their swings. Consequently, many teaching pros remove that distraction and teach the swing without the ball.

On the course, once you have relaxed, mentally rehearsed, physically rehearsed, and relaxed again, you must concentrate on the ball. You can "center" your attention on the back of the ball or even on a dimple on the ball.

Often great athletes don't remember what happened during a record-breaking performance. All they remember is their total concentration on a spot. This is as it should be in golf. Focus on a dimple on the ball, then let your body take care of the rest.

This is such a simple concept, but the problem is that we forget to do it. The tennis player forgets to watch the ball and instead looks for an opening in the opposite court. The golfer hears a passing cart and forgets to focus on the ball. Ideally, your concentration should be so intense that you don't even see the grass.

So there you have it. The simple steps that science has shown us will improve our games are: (1) mentally rehearse, (2) physically rehearse, (3) relax, and (4) concentrate on a center of focus. So simple, but each step requires practice to make it happen.

Summary

1. Since golf is a mental as well as a physical game, golfers must work to improve the mental side of their games as well as the physical.
2. Mental imagery (imagining what one will do) is an essential aspect of practice for golf, as it is for all other sports.
3. It is essential to learn how to relax before and during the golf swing.
4. Concentration on the ball is essential in executing an effective golf stroke.

16   *Nutrition for Better Health*

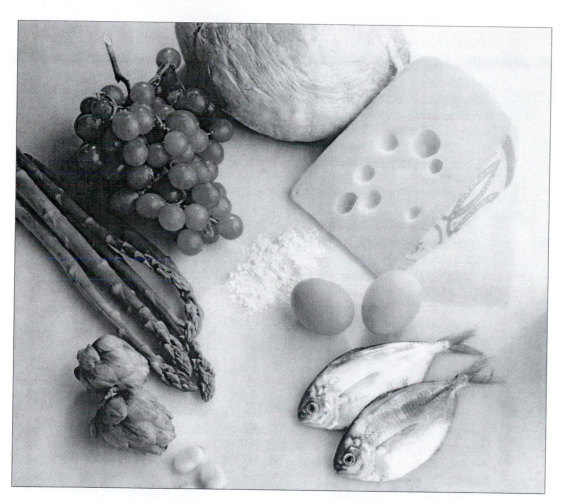

Outline

Along and full life requires exercise, an adequate diet, and play—both physical and mental—and a basic understanding of the science of nutrition is essential to healthy living. If you are going to play golf you will need adequate fuel for your athletic body. This chapter describes the basic elements of good nutrition. In the next chapter we will discuss how to apply these nutritional principles to your diet and weight management.

Nutrition

An informed person is aware of the nutrients necessary for minimal function, and can then put that knowledge into practice by developing a proper diet. Unfortunately, very few people consume even the minimum amounts of each of the necessary nutrients—protein, fat, carbohydrates, vitamins, minerals, and water (the essential nonnutrient). The first three nutrients listed (protein, fat, and carbohydrates) provide the energy required to keep us alive, in addition to making other specific contributions to our bodies.

The calorie measure used in counting food energy is really a kilocalorie—one thousand times larger than the calorie used as a measurement of heat in your chemistry class. In one food calorie (kilocalorie), there is enough energy to heat one kilogram of water one degree Celsius, or to lift 3,000 pounds of weight one foot high. So those little calories you see listed on cookie packages pack a lot of energy.

Most people need about 10 calories per pound of body weight just to stay alive. If you plan to do something other than just lie in bed all day, you probably need about 17 calories per pound of body weight per day in order to keep yourself going. And if you decide to play a couple of hours of singles, you can count on using a whole lot more calories.

Protein

Protein is made up of 22 *amino acids*, which consist of carbon, hydrogen, oxygen, and nitrogen. While both fats and carbohydrates contain the first three elements, nitrogen is found only in protein. Protein is essential for building nearly every part of the body—the brain, heart, organs, skin, muscles, and even the blood.

There are four calories in one gram of protein. Adults require 0.75 grams of protein per kilogram of body weight per day; this translates into one-third a gram of protein per pound. So an easy way to estimate your protein requirements in grams per day would be to divide your body weight by three. For instance, if you weigh 150 pounds, you need about 50 grams of protein per day.

Physically active adults have been thought to require more protein than is recommended by the United States Recommended Daily Allowance (USRDA), which is set at .8 grams per kilogram of body weight per day. In fact, most active people do not need to eat additional protein if 12 to 15 percent of their total calories is protein. Since active individuals need to consume more calories per day than their inactive counterparts due to their increased energy expenditure, active adults who keep their protein intake at around 15 percent of their total calories will eat more protein per day and thereby fulfill their body's protein requirement. Excess protein consumption (above the body's requirement) is broken down and the calories are either burned off or stored as fat.

However, when you are involved in a strenuous strength training regimen, as you might be if you play competitive golf, it may be necessary to increase your protein intake percentage, depending on the number of total calories you consume per day.

In order for your body to make any kind of tissue, including muscle, you must first have all of the necessary amino acids. Your body can manufacture some of them, while you must get others from your food. Those amino acids that you must get from your food are called the *essential amino acids*, while the others that you can make are known as the *nonessential amino acids*. During childhood, nine of the 22 amino acids are essential, while in adulthood we acquire the ability to synthesize one additional amino acid, leaving us with eight essential amino acids.

Amino acids cannot be stored in the body, so we need to consume our minimum amounts of protein every day. If adequate protein is not consumed, the body immediately begins to break down tissue (usually beginning with muscle tissue) to release the essential amino acids. If even one essential amino acid is lacking, the other essential ones are not able to work to their capacities. For example, if methionine (the most commonly lacking amino acid) is present at 60 percent of the minimum requirement, the other seven essential amino acids are limited to near 60 percent of their potential. When they are not used, amino acids are excreted in the urine.

Animal products (fish, poultry, and beef) and animal byproducts (milk, eggs, and cheese) are rich in readily usable protein. This means that when you eat animal products or by-products, the protein you consume can be converted into protein in your body because these sources have all of the essential amino acids in them. These foods are called *complete protein sources*.

Incomplete protein sources are any other food sources that provide protein but not all of the essential amino acids. Examples of incomplete proteins include peas and nuts. These food sources must be combined with other food sources that have the missing essential amino acids so that you can make protein in your body. Examples of complementary food combinations are rice and beans or peanut butter on whole wheat bread.

Another reason to be aware of complementary food combinations is that they enhance the absorption of the protein consumed. The person who is aware of the varying qualities of proteins can combine them to take advantage of the strengths of each. For example, if you eat flour at breakfast in the form of a piece of toast or coffee cake and wash it down with coffee, then drank a glass of milk at lunch, each of the protein sources would be absorbed by your body at a lower level. But if you ate bread with the milk at either meal, the higher protein values of both would be absorbed by your body immediately.

Fats

Fat is made of carbon, hydrogen, and oxygen. There are nine calories in a gram of fat. In the body, fat is used to develop the myelin sheath that surrounds the nerves. It also aids in the absorption of vitamins A, D, E, and K, which are the fat-soluble vitamins. It serves as a protective layer around our vital organs, and it is a great insulator against the cold. It is also a great concentrated energy source. And of course its most redeeming quality is that it adds flavor and juiciness to food!

Just as protein is broken down into different kinds of nitrogen compounds called amino acids, there are also different kinds of fats. There are three major kinds of fats, or fatty acids: saturated fats, monounsaturated fats, and polyunsaturated fats.

Saturated fats are "saturated" with hydrogen atoms. They are generally solid at room temperature and are most often found in animal fats, eggs, and whole milk products. Since these are the fats that are primarily responsible for raising the blood cholesterol level and hardening the arteries, they should be minimized in your diet.

Monounsaturated fats (oleic fatty acids) have room for two hydrogen ions to double-bond to one carbon. They are liquid at room temperature and are found in great amounts in olive, peanut, and canola (rapeseed) oils. Dietary monounsaturated fats have been shown to help the body excrete dietary cholesterol, thereby contributing a positive effect on atherosclerosis, one type of arteriosclerosis.

Polyunsaturated fats (linoleic fatty acids) have at least two carbon double bonds available, which translates into space for at least four hydrogen ions. Polyunsaturated fats are also liquid at room temperature and are found in the highest proportions in vegetable sources. Safflower, corn, and linseed oils are good sources of this type of fat. Polyunsaturated fatty acids of the omega-3 type may also contribute to the prevention of atherosclerosis.

We eat too much fat. The minimum requirement for fat in the diet is considered to be somewhere between 10 and 20 percent of the total calories consumed. The absolute maximum should be 30 percent, which is the amount now recommended for the American diet. While we as a society are still above this 30 percent value, we have been declining since the 1970s, and we need to keep that trend going. Most of us consume between 35 and 50 percent of our total calories in fats, with a very high percentage in saturated fats—the fats that we want to avoid.

Our high fat intake, most of which is saturated, tends to raise blood cholesterol levels in many people. If you are interested in decreasing the chances of developing hardened arteries by lowering your blood cholesterol level, it is recommended that you follow a diet low in fat (with the saturated fat intake at 10 percent or less of your total diet) and consume less than 300 milligrams of cholesterol daily. Or to put it another way, keep the total calories from fat under a third of your total intake and eat twice as much polyunsaturated and monounsaturated fat as saturated fat.

In the past, companies were allowed to identify the oil in a product on their labels as simply vegetable oil; under the Food and Drug Administration requirements made in 1976, they are now required to note whether it is corn oil, cottonseed oil, soybean oil, and so on, because some oils, even though they are not of animal origin, are very high in saturated fat. Palm kernel oil and coconut oil, often referred to as "tropical oils," are particularly high in saturated fats.

When you buy foods, especially cookies and crackers, always check the type of fat used. Avoid those with palm kernel oil and coconut oil. Also be aware of the hydrogenated oils used. While a hydrogenated safflower or canola oil may still have an acceptable fat ratio, a hydrogenated peanut or cottonseed oil may not contain the desired levels of unsaturated fats. Partially hydrogenated vegetable oils may contribute to the development of heart disease. The dietary use of hydrogenated corn oil stick margarine has been shown to increase LDL cholesterol levels when compared to the use of similar amounts of corn oil, also indicating an increased risk of heart disease.

In terms of controlling one's blood cholesterol level, dietary cholesterol is not as important as saturated fats in your diet. For this reason, saturated fats such as red meats, butter, egg yolks, chicken skin, and other animal fats should be greatly decreased. As an informed consumer, you may want to keep track of both your total fat intake and your intake of saturated fat to become better aware of your potential risk for heart disease. For example, one egg contains 5.6 grams of fat and only 0.7 grams of polyunsaturated fat, while an equal weight of hamburger contains 8.7 grams of fat and only 0.4 grams of polyunsaturated fats.

Carbohydrates

Carbohydrates are made from carbon, hydrogen, and oxygen, just as are fats, but "carbs" are generally a simpler type of molecule. There are four calories in a gram of carbohydrate. If carbohydrates are not utilized as immediately for energy as sugar (glucose), they are either stored in the body as glycogen (the stored form of glucose) or synthesized into fat and stored. Some carbohydrates cannot be broken down by the body's digestive processes; these are called fibers and will be discussed later. Digestible carbohydrates, can be separated into two categories: simple and complex. *Simple carbohydrates* are the most readily usable energy source in the body and include such things as sugar, honey, and fruit. *Complex carbohydrates* are the starches, which also break down into sugar for energy, but their breakdown is slower than with simple "carbs." Complex carbohydrates also bring with them various vitamins and minerals.

People in the United States often eat too many simple carbohydrates. These are often referred to as "empty calories," because they have no vitamins, minerals, or fibers. While a person who uses a great deal of energy can consume these empty calories without potential weight gain, most of us find these empty calories settling on our hips. The average person consumes 125 pounds of sugar per year, which is equivalent to one teaspoon every 40 minutes, night and day. Since each teaspoon of sugar contains 17 calories, this amounts to 231,000 calories or 66 pounds of potential body fat if this energy is not used as fuel for daily living.

High-carbohydrate diets that are especially high in sugar may be hazardous to one's health. They can increase the amount of triglycerides produced in the liver. These triglycerides are blood fats and are possible developers of hardened arteries. Also, a diet high in simple carbohydrates can lead to obesity, which can then result in the development of late-onset diabetes.

Fiber

Fiber is that part of the foods we take in that is not digestible. Fiber helps to move food through the intestines by increasing their peristaltic action. Vegetable fibers are made up chiefly of cellulose, an indigestible carbohydrate that is the main ingredient in the cell walls of plants. Plant-eating animals, such as cows, can digest cellulose. Meat-eating animals, such as humans, do not have the proper enzymes in their digestive tracts to metabolize cellulose.

Bran—the husks of wheat, oats, rice, rye, and corn—is another type of fiber. Bran is indigestible because of the silica in the outer husks. Some fibers, such as wheat bran, are also insoluble. The major function of fiber is to add bulk to the feces and to speed digested foods through the intestines. This reduces one's risk of constipation, intestinal cancer, appendicitis, and diverticulosis.

Some types of fibers are soluble; that is, they can find and eliminate certain substances such as dietary cholesterol. Pectin, commonly found in raw fruits (especially apple skins), oat and rice brans, and some gums from the seeds and stems of tropical plants (such as guar and xanthin) are examples of soluble fibers that pick up cholesterols as they move through the intestines.

Foods high in fiber are also valuable in weight-reducing diets because when foods pass more quickly through the digestive tract, the time available for absorption is reduced. Fiber also cuts the amount of hunger experienced by a dieter because it fills the stomach. A large salad with a diet dressing might give you very few calories, but it contains enough cellulose to fill your stomach, cut hunger, and move other foods through the intestinal passage.

Food processing often removes natural fiber from our food, and this is one of the primary reasons that we in the western world have relatively low amounts of fiber in our diet. For instance, white bread has only a trace of fiber—about nine grams in a loaf—while old-fashioned whole wheat bread has 70 grams. And when you peel a carrot or an apple, you remove much of the fiber.

Dietitians urge us to include more fiber in our diets. People should be particularly conscious of the benefits of whole-grain cereals, bran, and fibrous vegetables. Root vegetables (carrots, beets, and turnips) and leafy vegetables are very good sources of fiber. The average American diet has between 10 and 20 grams of fiber in it per day. This low level of fiber is believed to account for the

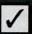 **Checklist for Effective Eating**

1. Eat 12 to 15 percent of your diet in proteins, preferably fish, fowl without skin, and beans.
2. Keep your fat intake between 10 and 30 percent of your total calorie intake, with saturated fat intake 10 percent or less and a higher proportion of monounsaturated fat.
3. Most of your diet should be complex carbohydrates (less-refined products) such as whole wheat, fruits, and vegetables.
4. It is recommended that people supplement with antioxidant vitamins (beta carotene, vitamins C and E).

fact that we have about twice the rate of colon cancer as do other countries whose citizens eat more fiber. This is why the National Cancer Institute has recommended that we consume between 25 and 35 grams of fiber per day.

Vitamins

Vitamins are organic compounds that are essential in small amounts for the growth and development of animals and humans. They act as enzymes (catalysts) that facilitate many of the body's processes. Although there is controversy about the effects of consuming excess vitamins, nutritionists agree that we need a minimum amount of vitamins for proper functioning.

Some vitamins are soluble only in water; others need fat to be absorbed by the body. The water-soluble vitamins, B complex and C, are more fragile than the fat-soluble vitamins, because they are more easily destroyed by the heat of cooking, and if they are boiled, they lose some of their potency into the water. Since they are not stored by the body, they should be included in the daily diet. However, even though they are not stored in the body, it is still possible to ingest too many water-soluble vitamins, leading to kidney stones because of the excess demand placed on the kidneys for processing.

The fat-soluble vitamins, A, D, E, and K, need oils in the intestines to be absorbed by the body. They are more stable than the water-soluble vitamins and are not destroyed by normal cooking methods. Because they are stored in the body, there is the possibility of ingesting too much of them—especially vitamins A and D.

Although nutritional researchers disagree about whether vitamin supplements are necessary, many of them see the necessity for supplementation with the vitamins that neutralize free oxygen radicals. Free oxygen radicals are harmful substances produced by many natural body processes, air pollution, and smoke, and seem to be responsible for some cancers and other diseases. Physical exercise, for all of its benefits, is one producer of free oxygen radicals.

Supplementation with antioxidants (beta carotene, vitamins C and E) reduces free oxygen radicals in the body. Dr. Ken Cooper, the man who coined the term "aerobics" and developed the first world-recognized fitness program, suggests a minimum supplementation of 400 IU of vitamin E, 1,000 mg of vitamin C, and 25,000 of beta carotene daily to counteract the potential damage done to the body by free oxygen radicals.

Minerals

Minerals are usually structural components of the body, but they sometimes participate in certain body processes. The body uses many minerals: phosphorus, calcium, and magnesium for strong teeth and bones; zinc for growth; chromium for carbohydrate metabolism; and copper and iron for hemoglobin production in the blood.

Iron is used primarily in developing hemoglobin, which carries oxygen in red blood cells. Women need more iron (18 milligrams a day) than men until they go through menopause, at which time their iron requirements drop to that of men (10 milligrams a day). Iron deficiency, common in women athletes, may impair athletic performance and should be corrected with supplementation.

Magnesium is the eighth most abundant element on the earth's surface. It seems to help activate enzymes essential to energy transfer. It is crucial for effective contraction of the muscles. Exercise depletes this element, so supplementation may be called for. When it is not present in sufficient amounts, twitching, tremors, and undue anxiety may develop.

Calcium is primarily responsible for building strong bones and teeth. For this reason, it seems obvious that a diet that is chronically low in calcium would have a negative effect on one's bone strength. Low calcium intake results in brittle and porous bones as one gets older, a condition known as osteoporosis. This is diagnosed when bone density shows a loss of 40 percent of the necessary calcium. It happens quite often in older people, especially women who have gone through menopause or have had their ovaries removed, because estrogen seems to protect against bone loss.

In teenage and young adult years, the inclusion of adequate calcium (which may be higher than the current Recommended Daily Allowance, or RDA) can aid in the development of peak bone mass, which can help prevent osteoporosis later on in life. Another contributing factor to osteoporosis is the imbalance of phosphorus to calcium in the typical diet. Calcium and phosphorous work together, and should be consumed on a one-to-one ratio. However, the average diet is much higher in phosphorus than calcium, leading to a leaching of calcium from the bones to make up for this imbalance.

Calcium is also necessary for strong teeth, nerve transmissions, blood clotting, and muscle contractions. Without enough calcium, muscle cramps often result. Skipping milk with its necessary calcium may be the cause of menstrual cramping for some girls. The uterus is a muscle, and muscles need both sodium and calcium for proper contractile functioning.

Phytochemicals

Phytochemicals (phyto is the Greek word for "plant") include thousands of chemical compounds that are found in plants. Some of these are vitamins and many have no known effect on us; however, more and more are being found to be highly beneficial.

In the past, the phytonutrients found in fruits and vegetables were classified as vitamins: Flavonoids were known as vitamin P, cabbage factors (glucosinolates and indoles) were called vitamin U, and ubiquinone was vitamin Q. Tocopherol somehow stayed on the list as vitamin E. The vitamin designation was dropped for other nutrients because specific deficiency symptoms could not be established. "Vita" means "life," so if the compound could not be found to be absolutely essential for life, it was dropped as a "vitamin," but is now classified as a phytochemical.

Various phytochemicals have been found to reduce the chance of cancers developing, reduce the chance of heart attack, reduce blood pressure, and increase immunity factors. Few of these have been reduced to pill form, such as vitamin pills, so they must be consumed in fruits and vegetables daily. It is suggested that each of us consume at least five servings of raw fruits or vegetables daily. Since many of the phytochemicals are heat sensitive, cooking can destroy some or all of the active ingredients.

We are a long way from developing highly effective phytochemical supplements, because there are so many elements and they may be destroyed in the processing. Garlic pills, for example, are available. However, in the deodorized versions, some active ingredients have been removed—they were in the chemicals that give garlic its "aroma."

Several types of phytochemicals are being studied. *Plant sterols* are somewhat similar to the animal sterol cholesterol but are unsaturated. These plant sterols compete for the same sites and thereby lower the blood cholesterol levels by as much as 10 percent. Soy is a good source for such sterols. Most green and yellow vegetables, and particularly their seeds, contain essential sterols.

Phenols have the ability to block specific enzymes that cause inflammation. They also modify the prostaglandin pathways and thereby protect blood platelets from clumping, thereby reducing the risk of blood clots. Blue, blue-red, and violet colorations seen in berries, grapes, and purple eggplant are due to their phenolic content.

Flavonoids is the name for a large group of compounds found primarily in tea, citrus fruits, onions, soy, and wine. Some can be irritating, but others seem to reduce heart attack risk. For example, the phenolic substances in red wine inhibit oxidation of human LDL cholesterol. The biologic activities of flavonoids include action against allergies, inflammation, free radicals, liver toxins, blood clotting, ulcers, viruses, and tumors.

Terpenes such as those found in green foods, soy products, and grains comprise one of the largest classes of phytonutrients. The most intensely studied terpenes are carotenoids—as evidenced by the many recent studies on beta carotene. Only a few of the carotenoids have the antioxidant properties of beta carotene. These substances are found in bright yellow, orange, and red plant pigments found in vegetables such as tomatoes, parsley, oranges, pink grapefruit, and spinach.

Limonoids are a subclass of terpenes found in citrus fruit peels. They appear to protect lung tissue and aid in detoxifying harmful chemicals in the liver.

Recent research confirms suspicion of the effects of soy products and related foods, which have long been used in Oriental diets. It has long been observed that Oriental women do not experience the problems of menopause, such as hot flashes, that western women commonly endure, but until recently, no theories have been advanced. Now we realize that a major factor is the fact that the Asians eat more vegetables, particularly soybeans.

It is phytoestrogens—plant chemicals that mimic the effects of the female hormone estrogen—that seem to be the major factor. These plant-like estrogens have similar effects to the natural estrogen in reducing heart disease, maintaining brain functions, reducing the incidence of breast cancer, and reducing softening of the bones (osteoporosis). In addition, other positive effects, which may or may not be related to estrogen intake, also occur, such as reduction in cancers (prostate, endometrial, bowel) and the effects of alcohol abuse[1].

Water

Water is called the essential nonnutrient because it has no nutritional value, yet without it we would die. Water makes up approximately 60 percent of the adult body, while an infant's body is nearly 80 percent water. Water cools the body through perspiration, carries nutrients to and waste products from the cells, helps cushion our vital organs, and is an essential element of all body fluids.

The body has about 18 square feet of skin that contains about 2 million sweat glands. On a comfortable day, a person perspires about a half-pint of water. Somebody exercising on a severely hot day may lose as much as seven quarts of water. If this is not replaced, severe dehydration can result. It is therefore generally recommended that we daily drink eight 8-ounce glasses of water or the equivalent in other fluids. This amount is dependent on the climate in which you live, the altitude at which you live, the type of foods that you eat, and the amount of activity that you participate in on a day-to-day basis. Golf can be strenuous and makes us sweat—so be sure to drink plenty of water when you play.

---

[1] S. A. Bingham et al., "Phyto-oestrogens: Where are we now?" *British Journal of Nutrition*, May 1998, 79(5) 393–406; S. T. Willard and L. S. Frawley, ""Phytoestrogens have agonistic and combinatorial effects on estrogen-responsive gene expression in MCF-7 human breast cancer cells," *Endocrinology*, April 1998, 8(2), 117–121; T. B. Clarkson, "The potential of soybean phytoestrogens for postmenopausal hormone replacement therapy," *Proceedings of the Society of Experimental Biological Medicine*, March 1998, 217(3), 365–368.

Summary

1. The basic macronutrients are proteins, fats, and carbohydrates.

2. Proteins are made of amino acids. Eight of these are considered to be essential and should be consumed daily.

3. Our bodies need fats, but they should be limited to 10 to 20 percent of our daily calorie intake.

4. Saturated fats and cholesterol are risk factors for heart disease.

5. The greatest percentage of our diets should be in complex carbohydrates, which contain vitamins, minerals, and fiber.

6. While proteins, fats, and carbohydrates (macronutrients) provide most of the nutrients we consume, the micronutrients (vitamins, minerals, and phytochemicals) are also essential.

7. Vitamins break down macronutrients and accomplish other essential body functions.

8. Free oxygen radicals are harmful byproducts of living that can be reduced by some vitamins (beta carotene, vitamins C and E).

9. Minerals are necessary building blocks of the body and are essential in all tissue.

10. Phytochemicals are desirable—and possibly necessary—elements found in plants, and may aid us in obtaining a higher level of nutrition.

11. Vitamin supplementation may be necessary for many people; most of us apparently profit from antioxidant supplementation.

12. Water is essential to all the body's functions; eight glasses of water a day are recommended.

17 *Sensible Eating and Weight Management*

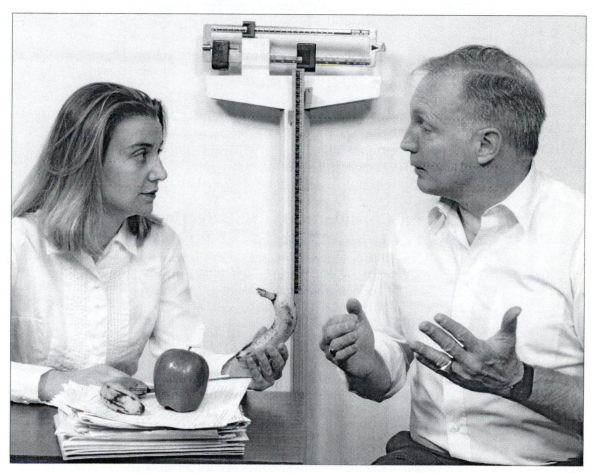

Outline

To eat sensibly, you must understand the basic principles of nutrition discussed in Chapter 16. Necessary nutrients must occur in your diet in proper quantities, and the calories you consume must be the amount necessary in order to maintain your desired weight. If you don't maintain your optimal weight, you may develop obesity and the diseases associated with obesity, such as diabetes, high blood pressure, and heart disease.

There are other factors that the sensible eater must understand. Caloric needs change according to climate and the amount of activity in which the person participates. For example, hot weather necessitates a greater intake of fluids due to the loss of water through perspiration, and you need fewer calories because your body does not need to burn as many calories to maintain its 98.6° Fahrenheit temperature.

A person using a great many calories, such as an active golf player, needs more carbohydrates, but it is a myth that athletes need a great deal more protein than non-athletes. While caloric needs may nearly double for the athlete who is expending a great deal of energy, protein needs are increased only slightly—usually less than 30 percent.

Important Considerations in Selecting Your Diet

The U.S. Department of Agriculture has devised a suggested diet guide called the Food Guide Pyramid. Its base is grain products, next comes fruits and vegetables, then meats and animal products, and at the top some fats or sweets if needed. There are six food groups in the pyramid:

- Grain products (breads, cereals, pastas): six to eleven servings per day recommended

- Vegetables: three to five servings per day recommended

- Fruits: two to four servings per day recommended

- High-protein meats and meat substitutes (meat, poultry, fish, beans, nuts, tofu/soy, eggs): two to three servings per day recommended

- Milk products: two servings per day for adults, three for children recommended

- Extra calories, if needed, from fats and/or sweets

Grain products provide the carbohydrates needed for quick energy. A serving size is one slice of bread, an ounce of dry cereal, or a half-cup of cooked cereal, pasta, or rice. Daily needs are six to eleven servings.

Grains are rich in B vitamins, some minerals, and fiber. Whole grains are the best sources of fibers. Refining grains or polishing rice reduces the fiber, the mineral content, and the B vitamins. This occurs in white and wheat bread (not whole wheat), pastas, pastries, and white rice. Flour is often refortified with three of the B complex vitamins, but seldom with the other essential nutrients.

If you want to reduce your cholesterol level, thereby reducing your chances of heart disease, reduce your chances of developing gallstones, or have a softer bowel movement, eat more of the soluble fibers (oat bran cereals, whole grain

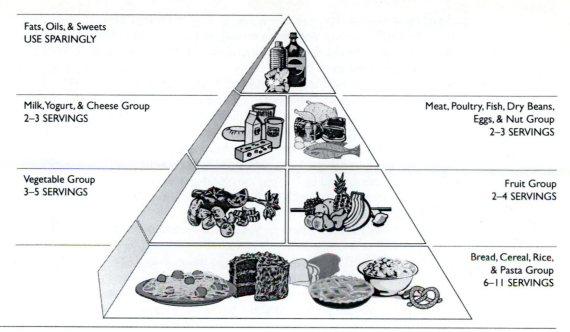

Fats, Oils, & Sweets
USE SPARINGLY

Milk, Yogurt, & Cheese Group
2–3 SERVINGS

Meat, Poultry, Fish, Dry Beans,
Eggs, & Nut Group
2–3 SERVINGS

Vegetable Group
3–5 SERVINGS

Fruit Group
2–4 SERVINGS

Bread, Cereal, Rice,
& Pasta Group
6–11 SERVINGS

The Food Guide Pyramid

bread with oats, rice bran, carrots, potatoes, apples, and citrus juices that contain pulp). If your concern is reducing your risk of intestinal cancers, appendicitis, and diverticulosis, eat more of the insoluble fibers (whole wheat breads and cereals, corn cereals, prunes, beans, peas, nuts, most vegetables, and polished rice).

Vegetables are rich in fibers, beta carotene, some vitamins, and minerals. Among the most nutritious vegetables are broccoli, carrots, peas, peppers, and sweet potatoes. If you are trying to lose weight, many vegetables are high in water and in fibers but low in calories. Among these are all greens (lettuce, cabbage, celery) as well as cauliflower. Actually, most vegetables are quite low in calories. You need three to five servings daily; a serving size is a half-cup of raw or cooked vegetables or a cup of raw leafy vegetables.

Fruits are generally high in vitamin C and fiber, and they are also relatively low in calories. You should have two to four servings daily; a serving size is one-fourth cup of dried fruit, a half-cup of cooked fruit, three-quarters cup of fruit juice, a whole piece of fruit, or a wedge of a melon.

Protein sources such as meats, egg whites, nuts, and beans are also high in minerals and vitamins B-6 and B-12. You need two to three servings a day; a serving is two and one-half ounces of cooked meat, poultry or fish, two egg whites, four tablespoons of peanut butter, one and one-fourth cups of cooked beans. A McDonald's "Quarter-Pounder" would give you two servings. The hidden eggs in cakes and cookies also count. The best meat products to eat are fish, egg whites, and poultry without the skin.

Red meat not only has a relatively low quality of protein (ranked after egg white, milk, fish, poultry, and organ meats), but it is linked to both cancers (two and a half times the risk for colon cancer) and heart disease. It also carries a great amount of fat, even if the fat on the outside is trimmed off. There is also a lot of cholesterol in the meat and fat of all land animals. Taking the skin off poultry greatly reduces the amount of fat and cholesterol that will be consumed, because poultry carry much of their fat next to the skin.

Of the animal proteins, fish has a higher quality of protein than meat or poultry. Also, fish are able to convert polyunsaturated linolenic fatty acids from plants they eat into omega-3 oils, which work to prevent heart disease by reducing cholesterol and by making the blood less likely to clot in the arteries. They do this by interfering with the body's production of the prostaglandin thromboxane, which increases blood clotting.

Milk and milk products (cheeses, yogurt, ice cream) are high in calcium and protein as well as in some minerals (potassium and zinc) and riboflavin. Adults need two servings daily, while children need three; a serving is one cup of milk or yogurt, one and one-half ounces of cheese, two cups of cottage cheese, one and one-half cups of ice cream, or one cup of pudding or custard.

Fats and sweets are positioned at the top of the pyramid of foods. They should be eaten only if a person needs extra calories. Consuming more fat than the recommended maximum of 30 percent of one's diet can be quite harmful— particularly in causing cancers and hardened arteries. Most researchers suggest a maximum of 10 to 20 percent of the diet in fats, with most in the form of monounsaturated and polyunsaturated fatty acids.

Sweets may assist in the development of tooth caries (cavities), but are not otherwise harmful if calories are not a problem for you. An athlete consuming 5,000 calories in a day can probably eat candy bars and ice cream, but the person attempting to control their weight should avoid them.

In addition to merely consuming the right proportions of foods, a concerned person would implement several other precautions:

- Avoid milk fat by drinking nonfat milk and milk products; eating ice milk (3 percent fat) or frozen desserts made without milk fat; and eating no-fat or low-fat cheeses. Half of the calories in whole milk come from the 3 ½ percent of the milk that is fat. Low-fat milk is reduced in fat calories by 40 percent. When low-fat milk is advertised as 98 percent fat-free, it is not that much better than whole milk, which is 96 ½ percent fat-free. The fats in milk are highly saturated—the worst kind of fat—yet the protein quality of milk is second only to egg whites.

- Avoid egg yolks because they contain a great deal of cholesterol and saturated fat. They are second only to caviar (fish eggs) in cholesterol content. Egg whites, on the other hand, have the highest rating for protein quality and are one of the best things you can eat.

- Reduce salt, because it is related to high blood pressure; and sugars, because they give "empty" calories—calories without other nutrients such as vitamins or fiber.

- Reduce fats to between 10 and 20 percent of your total calories. Normal salad dressings contain about 70 calories per tablespoon. If calories are a problem, use fat-free dressing or vinegar or lemon juice only. Rather than a butter or margarine, buy a good tasty whole-grain bread and eat it without grease. If you must use grease, use olive oil, or perhaps olive oil and balsamic vinegar as they serve in many Italian restaurants. If calories are not a concern and you like sweets, use jelly or jam.

- Never fry foods in oil; use a non-stick pan. If you must have an oil, use canola (rapeseed), olive, or safflower oil. Stay away from all fried foods, including potato chips. Fried foods not only add calories and saturated fats, but they also increase one's chances for intestinal cancers—as do all fats.

Beverages

Beverages make up a large part of our diet. We often don't think too much about the kinds of liquids we drink. The most nutritious drinks have been rated by the Center for Science in the Public Interest according to the amount of fat and sugar (higher content = lower rating), and their amount of protein, vitamins, and minerals (higher content = higher rating). Here are some sample results: skim or nonfat milk was rated +47, whole milk +38 (the lower rating was because of its fat content), orange juice +33, Hi-C +4, coffee 0, coffee with cream –1, coffee with sugar –12, Kool-Aid –55, and soft drinks –92.

Milk is the best beverage for most people. Children should have three to four cups each day, while adults should drink two cups. Our need for milk can be satisfied by other dairy products. For example, two cups of milk are equivalent to three cups of cottage cheese or five large scoops of ice cream. (Of course, this choice may *taste* the best, but there are obvious drawbacks to eating five scoops of ice cream every day!) In addition to its nutritional value as a developer of bones and organs, milk has been found to help people sleep. People who drink milk at night go to sleep more quickly, and sleep longer and sounder. This is because of the high content of the amino acid tryptophan, which makes serotonin, the neurotransmitter (brain chemical) associated with relaxation and calming.

Coffee contains several ingredients that may be harmful to the body. There are stimulants such as caffeine and the xanthines, as well as oils that seem to stimulate the secretion of excess acid in the stomach. And there are diuretics that eliminate water and some nutrients, such as calcium, from the body. Even two cups a day increases the risk of bone fractures[1]. A factor that may add to the risk of bone fractures is that people who drink more coffee usually drink little or no milk.

---

[1] E. Barrett-Connor, "Caffeine and bone fractures," *Journal of the American Medical Association*, January 26, 1994.

Caffeine is found in coffee, tea, and cola and many other drinks. Brewed coffee contains 100 to 150 milligrams of caffeine per cup (mg/cup), instant coffee about 90 mg/cup, tea between 45 and 75 mg/cup, and cola drinks from 40 to 60 mg/cup. Decaffeinated coffee is virtually free of caffeine, containing only two to four mg/cup. The therapeutic dose of caffeine given to people who have overdosed on barbiturates is 43 milligrams. Yet a cup of coffee contains up to 150 milligrams of caffeine!

Caffeine is a central nervous system stimulant. It elevates your blood pressure and constricts your blood vessels, both of which effects may assist in the development of high blood pressure. It has also been reported that excess caffeine in coffee, tea, and cola drinks can produce the same symptoms found in someone suffering from psychological anxiety, including nervousness, irritability, occasional muscle twitching, sensory disturbances, diarrhea, insomnia, irregular heartbeat, a drop in blood pressure, and occasionally failures of the blood circulation system.

Coffee is an irritant. The oils in coffee irritate the lining of the stomach and the upper intestines. People who drink two or more cups of coffee per day increase their chances of getting ulcers by 72 percent over non–coffee drinkers. Decaffeinated coffee is no more soothing to the ulcer patient than the regular blend, because both types increase the acid secretions in the stomach. Since an ulcer patient's acid secretion is not as high when caffeine alone is ingested (when compared to the acid levels after the ingestion of decaffeinated coffee), some other ingredient in coffee is thought to be responsible for these increased stomach acid levels.

Tea is not as irritating as coffee, but it does contain some caffeine and tannic acid, which can irritate the stomach. If you drink large amounts of tea, you should either take it with milk to neutralize the acid or add ice to dilute it. Green tea, the type commonly drunk in Asia, contains polyphenols, which appear to be antioxidants and may reduce cancer incidence. Black tea, the kind commonly drunk in Europe and America, has less of these protective substances[2]. Not much is known about the effects of herbal teas.

Alcohol contains seven calories per gram. These calories contain no nutritional elements, but they do contribute to your total caloric intake. Since alcoholic drinks are surprisingly high in calories, they contribute to the overweight problems of many individuals. People who drink alcoholic beverages and eat a balanced diet will probably consume too many calories. If they drink but cut down on eating, they may not develop a weight problem, but they will probably develop nutritional deficiencies that can result in severe illness. Alcohol is also a central nervous system depressant, which causes a decrease in one's metabolism.

---

[2] *University of California, Berkeley Wellness Letter*, January 1992, pp. 1–2.

In addition to the normal dangers of alcohol in creating alcoholism and destroying brain cells, there are other considerations in drinking. Beer or ale, because of their carbonation, have the effect of neutralizing stomach acid. This can increase the acids secreted by the stomach, causing ulcers.

Food Additives

Sugar is a negative for most people. In fact it is probably the most harmful additive to the foods that we in the United States eat. We average about 125 pounds of sugar per person per year. This gives us a lot of excess calories that, if not used for energy, will be stored as fat. As discussed previously, if we exceed our desired weight and become obese, we will have increased health risks.

Salt can be a dangerous food additive, yet most people do not consider adding salt to their food to be a health risk. But when you look at populations as a whole, it seems obvious that the higher the salt intake, the greater the frequency of high blood pressure.

Many manufacturers add salt to enhance the taste of food, and sodium is often high in processed or canned foods. While the desired intake is between one and two grams (1,000 and 2,000 milligrams), the average daily intake in America is five grams. The potential negative effect of a high sodium intake can be combated by ingesting a high level of potassium. However, the desired recommended daily allowance for potassium, 2.5 grams, is not met by the average American, who consumes only 0.8 to 1.5 grams daily. Most of our foods follow this same pattern—too high in sodium and too low in potassium.

Preservatives added to foods lengthen storage life and prevent disease-causing germs from multiplying. Most are harmless, and some give protection against intestinal cancers. Some, however, such as the nitrates in hot dogs, have been implicated in causing cancer. Nevertheless, the disease of botulism, which they prevent, is far more of a danger than that posed by the nitrates.

Vitamins and minerals have been added to food for years. In 1973, the Food and Drug Administration suggested that more iron be added to enrich flour after they found that iron is often low in our diets. Vitamins A and D are added to skim milk to make it nonfat milk—milk that has all of the nutrients of whole milk but without the fat. Vitamins A and D are fat soluble and stay in the fat when it is removed to make skim milk.

Vegetarianism

When vegetarians are careful about their dietary intakes, they may prove to be healthier than nonvegetarians. One study comparing healthy vegetarians to nonvegetarians found that healthy vegetarians had lower blood sugar and cholesterol levels than did their closely matched nonvegetarian counterparts.

Smart Shopping

Shopping for low-fat foods requires a sharp eye. If you are looking for a low-fat food, look at the total grams of fat, multiply by nine (nine calories per gram of fat), then divide that by the total number of calories in the food. (For example, if a food has three grams of fat, nine times that equals 27 total calories from fat. If the food has a total of 270 calories, then the percentage of fat calories is 10 percent.) If the food has one of the new food labels, it will list both the number of fat values and the approximate percentage of fat calories per serving. You want to keep your daily total percentage of fat below 30 percent to decrease your risk of developing heart disease. Even better than the suggested maximum of 30 percent is keeping the total to 10 or 20 percent fat.

Many foods, particularly low-fat liquids such as salad dressings without oil, have replaced the oil with some gums. Guar, locust bean, and xanthine gums are soluble fibers that help remove cholesterol from the intestines. So you get a double advantage—no fat and some cholesterol-removal substances.

The food label lists ingredients according to their content in the product. The higher on the list of ingredients, the more of that item is present in the food. So if the product lists wheat flour first, there is no problem. But if it lists eggs or hydrogenated oils second, the food may be too high in fat. And if you are watching your sodium intake, remember to look for salt on the list.

Eating and Overeating

People eat to nourish their bodies. But in America many people eat to reduce stress. We may not be satisfied in our work, at school, or in our relationships, but we can be satiated with food. Filling our stomachs can make us feel that in at least one part of our lives we are totally satisfied. When we eat to relieve stress, we will probably take in more calories than we need for living—but even worse, stress eating often means junk foods. It is much more intelligent to play some tennis to relieve stress.

Being overweight is a more common concern than is being underweight. While some people are overweight, some are obese. For example, 35 percent of women are 20 percent overweight.[3] Of people who are obese, one in 20 has a genetic factor or a problem in physical malfunctioning, such as an underactive thyroid, a problem with the hypothalamus, or one of the other centers of the brain that deals with whether or not we feel full or hungry. There are medical procedures that can help these people. In cases where the metabolism is slowed, such as by an underactive thyroid gland, doctors can administer the proper hormone to increase metabolism back into what is considered a normal range.

---

[3] *Harvard Women's Health Watch*, November 1994, p. 4.

Another cause of obesity is thought to be the number of fat cells in a person's body. This is known as the *set point theory*. It is thought that the more fat cells one has, the more one is driven to eat to maintain these fat cells. The number of fat cells one has is generally set after puberty.

For others, obesity is caused by overeating to an extreme degree. However, according to the Harvard University Nutrition Department, most people are overfat because they don't exercise, not because they overeat. Overeating coupled with a lack of exercise is a sure way to become obese.

Since it is the amount of body fat that a person carries that is the true culprit of disease, it is preferable to refer to this health risk as being overfat rather than being overweight. Many bodybuilders may be overweight when compared to the height/weight charts commonly used to measure health risks by insurance companies, but they are not overfat.

Determining if you are overfat can be done in several ways. The most common method is to look at yourself in a mirror. If you look fat, you may be fat. Another way is to pinch the fat you carry just below the skin. If you can pinch an inch, you are probably carrying too much fat. Professionals often use skin calipers to measure the amount of fat people carry in four to seven designated spots on the body, or they use underwater weighing or bioelectrical impedence.

Once your body fat percentage is determined, you can then find out what a healthy weight would be for you. Men are usually considered healthy if their body fat is in the range of 10 to 15 percent, while women are healthy if they fall between 18 to 25 percent body fat. Men are considered overfat if their body fat is over 20 percent, while women are overfat if their body fat is over 30 percent. Women require more fat than men do because of their menstrual cycle. If a woman falls below 12 percent body fat, she may become amenorrheic (lose her regular menstrual cycle).

Should You Lose Weight?

Before you decide to lose weight, you first need to determine whether your are overweight due to being overfat. From a health point of view, it is your proportion of fat and lean body mass that is most important.

How to Lose Weight

The wisest approach to losing weight would be to find out why you are overweight. If it is genetic, perhaps medical help is needed. If you eat because of stress, you should find another way to relieve stress, such as exercise or relaxation techniques or, if you must have something in your mouth, try gum or a low-calorie food. If your problem is a lack of exercise, start an effective exercise program. If you consume too many calories, you will need to change your diet.

Don't even start a weight-loss program if you are not willing to make lifestyle changes for the rest of your life. The great majority of dieters refuse to make such a commitment. That is why 40 percent of women and 25 percent of men are on a diet at any one time and the average American goes on 2.3 diets a year, and it is also why 95 percent of dieters regain all of their lost weight within five years. The average diet is just not successful.

In all likelihood, if you adopt the habits of effective exercise and a low-fat and low-alcohol eating pattern, the pounds will drop off. Losing weight just for the sake of being thinner seldom works for very long. You have to determine whether you honestly want a healthier lifestyle or just to look better for the summer. A pattern of continually gaining and losing weight is frustrating and probably not worth the effort. But a true lifestyle change to healthy eating and regular exercise will pay many mental, physical, and social dividends.

We must recognize that the fat we wear comes primarily from the fat we eat. Because carbohydrates are so efficiently converted to sugar glucose, they are used first for energy in the body. To convert carbohydrates to fat, about 23 percent of the energy is used to make the conversion. Protein, if not used, will normally be converted into sugars and will be the second source of available energy. But the fat you eat uses only 3 percent of its food value in the conversion to body fat.

So 25 grams of carbohydrate, which will yield 100 calories (at 4 calories a gram), is reduced by 23 percent of the calories used to convert them to body fat. But fats consumed in your food are different. Eleven grams of fat (at nine calories per gram) is 99 calories, but it only takes 3 percent of those calories to convert it all to body fat, and 96 calories of body fat can be deposited. So 100 calories of carbohydrates, if not used for energy, will become about 8.5 grams of body fat, but 100 calories of fat from the diet will become about 10.75 grams of body fat.

To lose one pound of fat per week, you must have a net deficit of 500 calories per day; one pound of fat contains 3,500 calories. You may choose to achieve this solely by decreasing your food intake by 500 calories per day.

You could also choose to increase your activity level to burn off 500 calories a day. Keep in mind that it takes a great deal of energy to achieve this goal, and it can be dangerous for you to embark on such a strenuous exercise program if you are not currently exercising. It is best to combine calorie reduction with exercise to achieve your goal. Aerobic exercise will keep your metabolism up as you lose the fat, and you won't have to restrict your calories as much because you will be burning off energy each time you exercise.

We now know that calories are used both during and after exercise. The longer and more vigorous the exercise, the longer one's metabolism is increased, so that for more hours after the exercise is completed, the calorie expenditure will be increased over normal. While this increase in calories burned after one has finished exercising is not a large amount, it is still an increase over one's resting metabolism, and a calorie burned is a calorie burned!

Some people think that exercising will make them eat more. A quarter-mile to a mile of jogging or a good set of tennis games will have no measurable

Calories Burned with Various Activities

	Calories per pound per hour	Calories expended by 150 lb. person in 20 minutes
Sleeping	0.36	18.0
Sitting at rest	0.55	27.5
Sitting at work	0.60	30.0
Light exercise (housework)	1.00	50.0
Walking	1.20	60.0
Jogging (slow)	1.75	87.5
Volleyball (recreational 6-person)	1.50	65.0
Golf	2.00	100.0

effect on the total intake of calories. In fact, by exercising just before a meal, you can dull your appetite and decrease your desire for more calories.

Eating Disorders

Anorexia nervosa is starvation by choice. This is a disease primarily seen in young women. It afflicts nearly one in a hundred women, although 5 to 10 percent of its victims are male. In this disease, the person goes on a diet and refuses to stop, no matter how thin he or she gets. About one out of ten people who have this disorder end up starving themselves to death. The disease has a psychological basis, but its physical effects are very real. Medical care, usually hospitalization, is generally required.

After the anorexic begins the severe dieting routine, symptoms of starvation may set in, leading to a number of physical problems. Abnormal thyroid, adrenal, and growth hormone functions are not uncommon. The heart muscle becomes weakened. Amenorrhea occurs in women and girls due to the low percentage of body fat. Blood pressure may drop. Anemia is common due to the lack of protein and iron ingested. The peristalsis of the intestines may slow and the lining of the intestines may atrophy. The pancreas often becomes unable to secrete many of its enzymes. Body temperature may drop. The skin may become dry and there can be an increase of body hair in the body's attempt to keep itself warm. And for 10 percent of sufferers, the result is death.

Because dieting is such a common occurrence in our society, anorexia is often difficult to diagnose until the person has entered the advanced stages of the disease. However, other symptoms such as moodiness, being withdrawn, obsessing about food but never being seen eating it, and constant food preparation may be observed by those close to the anorexic. Once diagnosed, there are a number of medical and psychological therapies that can be effective.

Bulimia, or *bulimia nervosa*, is more common than anorexia. The person with bulimia restricts calorie intake during the day, but binges on high-fat, high-calorie foods at least twice a week. Following the binge, the person purges in an attempt to get rid of the excess calories just consumed. Purging techniques include vomiting, laxatives, fasting, and excessive exercise. Some experts do not consider the behavior bulimic until it has persisted for about three months with two or more binges per week during that time. Estimates based on various surveys of college students and others indicate that between 5 and 20 percent of women may be bulimic. It is also more common among men than is anorexia.

Bulimia, like anorexia, stems from a psychological problem. However, in some cases there may also be a link to physical abnormalities. The neurotransmitters serotonin and norepinephrine seem to be involved, as does the hormone cholecystokinin, which is secreted by the hypothalamus and makes a person feel that enough food has been eaten.

Physical symptoms to look for depend on the type of purging technique used. The bulimic who induces vomiting can have scars on the back of the knuckles, mouth sores, gingivitis, tooth decay, a swollen esophagus, and chronic bad breath. The bulimic who uses laxatives has constant diarrhea, which can cause irreparable damage to the intestines. All bulimics run the risk of throwing off their electrolytes (minerals involved in muscle contractions) as a result of constant dehydration. It is this imbalance of electrolytes that can cause the bulimic to have abnormal heart rhythms and that can induce a heart attack.

Female athletes sometimes develop problems called the "female athletic triad,"[4] or a combination of eating disorders, osteoporosis, and amenorrhea. It is caused by the hard training practiced by competitive athletes or dancers and the desire to keep weight low, which often results in inadequate nutrition. Weight loss is sometimes achieved by bulimic methods. The result is weight that is too low, a loss of calcium from the bones, and a lack of healthy menstruation.

These problems are most likely to occur in activities in which low weight is an advantage, such as dancing, distance running, figure skating, and gymnastics, and it is more prevalent among athletes in individual sports than in team sports. Males, with the exception of competitive wrestlers, do not often experience the need to eat less.

---

[4] Aurelia Nattiv, Barbara Drinkwater, et al. "The female athletic triad," *Clinics in Sports Medicine: The Athletic Woman*, W. B. Saunders: Philadelphia, 13(2), April 1994, pp. 405–418.

Summary

1. Sensible eating requires some understanding of the science of nutrition.
2. Following the guidelines of the Food Pyramid will generally give a person an adequate diet.
3. Skim or nonfat milk is the best beverage.
4. Salt and sugar are the most common food additives.
5. Many people overeat and become overfat.
6. Most overfat people can lose weight through an effective diet and adequate exercise.
7. Eating disorders seem to be prevalent; anorexia nervosa and bulimia are the major eating disorders.

Self-Test

Write in the number that best describes your eating habits:

3—Almost always   2—Sometimes   1—Almost never

____ 1. Do you eat three or more pieces of fruit per day? (Fruit juice counts as one piece.)
____ 2. Do you eat a minimum of three servings of vegetables each day—including a green leafy or orange vegetable?
____ 3. Do you eat three or four milk products (such as milk, cheese, yogurt) per day?
____ 4. Do you eat a minimum of six servings of grain products (breads, cereal, pasta) each day?
____ 5. Do you eat breakfast?
____ 6. Do you eat fish at least three times per week?
____ 7. Do you avoid fried foods, including potato chips and french fries?
____ 8. Do you eat fast food fewer than three times per week?
____ 9. Are the milk products you consume made from nonfat milk?
____10. Do you avoid high-sugar foods and highly refined carbohydrates such as sweet rolls, cookies, nondiet sodas, candy, etc.?

Your Score
25–30   You are balancing your diet well.
18–24   Your diet needs to be improved.
10–17   Your diet is unhealthy.

Bulimia Self-Test

Write "Never," "Sometimes," or "Often" to describe your weight-control practices:

____ 1. Is your life a series of constant diets?

____ 2. Do you vomit or take laxatives or diuretics to control your weight?

____ 3. Do you alternate periods of eating binges with fasts to control your weight?

____ 4. Does your weight fluctuate by as much as 10 pounds because of eating habits?

____ 5. Have you ever had a "food binge" during which you ate a large amount of food in a short period of time?

____ 6. If you "binged," was it on high-calorie food such as ice cream, cookies, donuts, or cake?

____ 7. Have you ever stopped a binge by vomiting, sleeping, or experiencing pain?

____ 8. Do you think your eating habits vary from the average person's?

____ 9. Are you out of control with your eating habits?

____10. Are you close to 100 pounds overweight because of your eating habits?

If you marked two or more of the above questions "Often," you may have a serious eating disorder called *bulimia*.

Where to Go for Help

Anorexia Bulimia Treatment Education Center: 800-33-ABTEC

Bulimia Anorexia Self-Help: 800-227-4785

Low-fat diet gourmet meals are possible. Send for the free *Metropolitan Cookbook*. Write to: Health and Welfare Department, Metropolitan Life Insurance Co., 1 Madison Avenue, New York, NY 10010) . Or buy the American Heart Association's cookbook.

Height and Weight Table: Men*

Height	Small Frame	Medium Frame	Large Frame
5'2"	128–134	131–141	138–150
5'3"	130–136	133–143	140–153
5'4"	132–138	135–145	142–156
5'5"	134–140	137–148	144–160
5'6"	136–142	139–151	146–164
5'7"	138–145	142–154	149–168
5'8"	140–148	145–157	152–172
5'9"	142–151	148–160	155–176
5'10"	144–154	151–163	158–180
5'11"	146–157	154–166	161–184
6'0"	149–160	157–170	164–188
6'1"	152–164	160–174	168–192
6'2"	155–168	164–178	172–197
6'3"	158–172	167–182	176–202
6'4"	162–176	171–187	181–207

*Weights at ages 25 to 59 based on lowest mortality. Weight in pounds according to frame (in indoor clothing weighing 5 lbs.; shoes with 1" heels).
Source: 1999 Metropolitan Life Insurance Company height and weight tables.

Height and Weight Table: Women†

Height	Small Frame	Medium Frame	Large Frame
4'10"	102–111	109–121	118–131
4'11"	103–113	111–123	120–134
5'0"	104–115	113–126	122–137
5'1"	106–118	115–129	125–140
5'2"	108–121	118–132	128–143
5'3"	111–124	121–135	131–147
5'4"	114–127	124–138	134–151
5'5"	117–130	127–141	137–155
5'6"	120–133	130–144	140–159
5'7"	123–136	133–147	143–163
5'8"	126–139	136–150	146–167
5'9"	129–142	139–153	149–170
5'10"	132–145	142–156	152–173
5'11"	135–148	145–159	155–176
6'0"	138–151	148–162	158–179

†Weights at ages 25 to 59 based on lowest mortality. Weight in pounds according to frame (in indoor clothing weighing 3 lbs.; shoes with 1" heels).
Source: 1999 Metropolitan Life Insurance Company height and weight tables.

Appendix

Golf Resources

Rules of Golf

For the official rules of golf and additional information, contact:

United States Golf Association
P.O. Box 708
Far Hills, NJ 07931
Voice: 908-234-2300
Fax: 908-234-9687
Web: http://www.usga.org

Books About Golf

The following titles are a small sampling of the hundreds of books that have been written about golf. In addition to looking for golf books at your library or local bookstores, you can buy many golf titles online at either www.amazon.com or www.barnesandnoble.com.

Bailey, Bill. *Golf Etiquette 101.* Prima Publishing, 1998.

Borgenicht, David, Editor. *Golf: Great Thoughts on the Grand Game.* Running Press, 1995.

Celsi, Teresa Noel. *Golf: The Lore of the Links.* Andrews McMeel Publishing, 1992.

Chang, Cindy (Compiler). *Golf: Words from the Green.* Andrews McMeel Publishing, 1995.

Concannon, Dale. *Golfing Bygones.* Shire Publications, 1999.

Conner, Floyd. *Golf! Great Moments and Dubious Achievements in Golf History.* Chronicle Books, 1992.

Dorsel, Tom. *The Complete Golfer.* Allyn & Bacon, 1996.

Durbin, William. *Arnold Palmer (Golf Legends).* Chelsea House, 1998.

Feinstein, John. *A Good Walk Spoiled: Days and Nights on the PGA Tour.* Little Brown, 1996.

Gilbert, Thomas W. *Lee Trevino.* Chelsea House, 1992.

Foston, Paul (Editor). *The Encyclopedia of Golf Techniques: The Complete Step-by-Step Guide to Mastering the Game of Golf.* Running Press, 1994.

Garrity, John, and Bill Jaspersohn. *Sports Illustrated Putting: The Stroke-Saver's Guide.* Sports Illustrated, 1992.

Hobbs, Michael, and M. Hobbs. *Golf in Art.* Book Sales, 1996.

Hull, Mary. *The Composite Guide to Golf.* Chelsea House, 1998.

Gutman, Bill. *Tiger Woods: Golf's Shining Young Star.* Millbrook, 1998.

Kramer, Jon, and Jim Kramer. *Lee Trevino: Overcoming the Odds.* Raintree/Steck Vaughn, 1996.

McCord, Gary, et al. *Golf for Dummies.* IDG Books, 1999.

Mulvoy, Mark. *Sports Illustrated Golf: Play Like a Pro.* Sports Illustrated, 1994.

Murray, Bill, and George Peper. *Cinderella Story: My Life in Golf.* Doubleday, 1999.

Nicklaus, Jack, and Ken Bowden. *Jack Nicklaus' Lesson Tee.* Fireside, 1998.

Palmer, Mike. *Systematic Golf: A Complete Golf Instruction Course.* Sterling, 1993.

Penick, Harvey. *Harvey Penick's Little Red Book.* Fireside, 1999.

Peper, George (Editor). *Golf in America: The First One Hundred Years.* Abradale Press, 1994.

Rotella, Bob, and Bob Cullen. *Golf Is Not a Game of Perfect.* Simon & Schuster, 1995.

Rotella, Bob, and Bob Cullen. *The Golf of Your Dreams.* Simon & Schuster, 1997.

Snead, Sam, with Al Stump. *The Education of a Golfer.* Simon & Schuster, 1962.

Sports Illustrated (Editor). *Golf: Four Decades of Sports Illustrated's Finest Writing on the Game of Golf.* Sports Illustrated, 1996.

Updike, John. *Golf Dreams: Writings on Golf.* Fawcett Books, 1997.

Ward, Andrew. *Golf's Strangest Rounds.* Parkwest Publications, 1993.

Wheeler, Jill C. *Tiger Woods: Lion on the Links.* Abdo & Daughters, 1996.

Golf Internet Sites

There are thousands of golf-related Internet sites. They come and go. You can get everything from golf instruction to discounted equipment. The list that follows is not exhaustive, but will start your Internet search. You can find more sites by doing key word searches.

Golf Ball Warehouse
www.myballs.com
A great source of inexpensive golf balls. New and used balls from $5 a dozen up. Prices are even cheaper if you buy six dozen at a time. If you don't have access to the Internet, call 800-372-2557.

GolfWeb
http://services.golfweb.com
"Everything golf." A comprehensive, helpful site, with a great classifieds section.

GolfSearch
www.golfsearch.com
The great golf search engine; you can surf this wave forever!

FantasyTeam Sports
http://pga.fantasyteam.com
A weekly golf pool, with a prize to the winner. Great fun!

Yahoo's Golf Links
http://st3.yahoo.com
Search the online world of golf with the popular Yahoo directory!

Glossary

Ace A hole in one.

Addressing the ball Getting into your stance and getting ready to hit the ball.

Approach shot The shot you make from the fairway area to the green.

Apron The area surrounding the green that has longer grass than the grass on the green but shorter than the fairway grass.

Away Being farther away from the flag, so having the right to make the next shot.

Back nine The second 9 holes of an 18-hole course.

Backspin A reverse spin on the ball that will make it stop quickly after it lands. The higher-numbered clubs give more backspin.

Banana ball A slice.

Bite When the ball stops because of the backspin.

Birdie A score of one under par for that hole.

Bogey A score of one over par for that hole.

Break The change of direction of a putted ball due to the slope of the green or the grain of the grass.

Bunker A sand trap.

Caddie A person who carries one's clubs and who can give advice on how to play a hole.

Casual water Water that should not be on the course. It may be a result of rain or lawn sprinklers.

Chip shot A short shot played to the green.

Cup The hole.

Divot A piece of turf that has been dislodged by a stroke. It should be replaced and tamped down.

Draw A shot that curves slightly to the left—not as sharp as a hook.

Duffer or dub A player who doesn't play well.

Eagle A score of two under par for that hole.

Fade A shot that curves slightly to the right (for right-handers)—not as sharp as a slice.

Fairway The mowed grass area between the tee and the putting green.

Fat shot A shot in which the clubhead strikes the ground before it hits the ball, resulting in a shorter shot.

Flagstick The pole that holds the flag that marks the hole.

Flat swing A swing that is more horizontal than the typical swing.

Fore The warning yelled to alert people that a shot may endanger them. It can be yelled before the shot to clear the way or after an errant shot that is in flight.

Foursome Four players playing together.

Grounding the club Touching the sole of the club to the ground before making a shot.

Handicap The average number of strokes above par that a player shoots. It is often used in tournaments to give all the players a chance to win.

Hazard Water or sand areas (bunkers).

Hole out To finish playing the hole.

Hook A sharp left-curving ball.

Honors The right to tee off first because of winning the previous hole.

L.P.G.A. Ladies Professional Golf Association.

Lateral water hazard Water on the side of the fairway.

Lie The position of the ball as it lies on the ground.

Loose impediments Objects such as pebbles, leaves, and twigs that can be moved to clear the way for a shot.

Low handicapper One who is a good golfer but does not average par.

Match play The form of competition scored by total number of holes won rather than total number of strokes for the round. The player with the lowest strokes for a hole wins the hole, and the winner of the match is the one who has won the most holes.

Mulligan An illegal second shot taken when a player is unhappy with the first shot played.

Nassau A scoring system in which one point is given to the player who wins the front 9 holes, a second point is given to the winner of the back 9 holes, and a third point is given to the winner of the full 18 holes.

Net The score in a tournament after the handicaps are subtracted from the "gross" score.

Obstruction An object on the course that was not designed into the course.

Open A tournament in which both professionals and amateurs can play.

Out nine or front nine The first nine holes of the course.

Out-of-bounds An area in which you are not allowed to play the ball. It is usually marked by stakes indicating that the area is out of bounds.

P.G.A. Men's Professional Golf Association.

Par The number of strokes that a good player should take for that hole. Holes may be 3-par, 4-par, or 5-par.

Pin high The ball is even with the pin or hole.

Pitch shot A high shot used for getting onto the green.

Provisional ball A second ball hit when the first may have been lost or out of bounds.

Pull A shot that goes to the left of where it was aimed.

Push A shot that goes to the right of where it was aimed.

Rough Areas of tall grass area near the mown fairway.

Sand trap A depressed area filled with sand; also called a bunker.

Scotch foursome Two teams of two players each with each team playing only one ball. The team members alternate hitting the ball.

Scratch golfer One who shoots close to par. His or her handicap is zero.

Shank A shot hit on the neck of the club.

Slice A shot that curves to the right.

Stroke play The form of competition scored by the total number of strokes played for the round.

Summer rules The ball must be played as it lies.

Tee area The area from which the first shot is taken for each hole.

Thin shot One in which the clubhead hits high on the ball without hitting the turf.

Topping the ball Hitting the top of the ball and causing it to roll rather than fly.

U.S.G.A. United States Golf Association. It is the governing body for golf in the United States.

Wedge A club with more loft than a 9-iron. Pitching wedges are specifically for pitching. Sand wedges are heavier and are made for playing from sand traps.

Whiff A complete miss of the ball.

Winter rules Rules at some clubs that allow you to move the ball to a better lie at certain times. Generally, the lie cannot be improved more than one club length.

Index

CPSIA information can be obtained
at www.ICGtesting.com
Printed in the USA
FFOW04n0112230414
4983FF